What Is Your

What and who are the reasons you change your health, and ultimately ⸺⸺ ⸺⸺ ⸺ ⸺⸺⸺ ⸺⸺⸺ these things and people are Your Why. In the blank squares below, attach photos of Your Why, the things and the people in your life that are your motivation for deciding to do this program.

The first photo needs to be of YOU and if that photo is the only one, that is more than enough!

My WHY

Picture of YOU

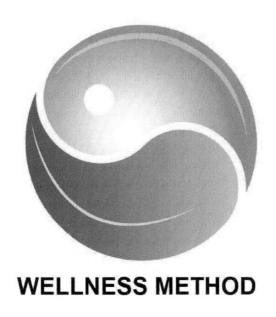

WELLNESS METHOD

Your Recreate 365

Success Journal

How to Master the Art and Science

to Recreate your Health and Recreate your Life.

YOUR DEDICATION PAGE

This book is dedicated to (write one or more names):

Dear,

1._____   2. _____

3. _____   4. _____

5. _____   6. _____

I am committed to working to improve myself so that I am healthier and managing stress more effectively so that I have more energy. This will allow me to do more of the things I want to do with you and better enjoy our time together. This will allow me to be more actively involved in LIFE so that I can be a better (circle all that apply):

Parent/s   *Spouse or Partner*   *Child/Children*

Teacher/s   *Role Model/s*   *Friend/s*

By improving my life, I hope to inspire others!

Sincerely,

_____
(your signature)

CONTENTS

INTRODUCTION

"When You Change the Way You Look at Things,
The Things You Look at Change."- Dr. Wayne Dyer

This quote by Dr. Wayne Dyer encapsulates a Wellness Mindset. It means that you alone decide how to interpret any situation or event in your life by the lens with which you choose to look through. Two people can experience the same exact challenging situation, but one may see it as a blessing and learn from it, while the other may see it as a big disaster and point fingers blaming others for it. If you are open to growing personally, you will find that many situations will become less and less of a challenge. When you learn how to appropriately respond you will begin to experience more joy in life.

Your beliefs about yourself, your friendships, romance, family, success, and spirituality, for instance, will dictate how your life plays out. Being open to change and growth means that every new experience you have, every book that you read, every new person you meet, and even a program like this can change your lenses of the world. As you evolve and change your life, your lenses will change accordingly. You can't control all the situations that occur in life, but you CAN control how your respond to them. Your THOUGHTS dictate your response.

As you move through your Recreate Program, you will notice that you are learning a lot! This learning is meant to challenge you so that your beliefs and thoughts will begin to work in your favor instead of against you. You will literally be Recreating your body, your thoughts, and your life during this program.

You are a miraculous being! In one year, you will automatically replace 98% of the cells within you. So, what about the remaining 2%? The remaining 2% are your brain cells! However, they will not automatically replace themselves like the rest of our body, so it's up to us to consciously work to rebuild and replace them. Since we are aware, and have studied this extensively at Wellness Method, we include Mindset work within your program so that you can Recreate your brain cells with the rest of your body! It is not as difficult as you might think- but as with any change, you must commit to it with your whole heart!

You Are in A Constant State of Recreation.

In one year, you will replace 98% of the cells in your body.

New stomach lining	5 days
New Skin	1 month
New DNA	6 weeks
New Red Blood Cells	3 months
New Liver	6 months
New Lungs	1 year

A GROWTH MINDSET

Time to buckle up and prepare to learn and grow as you RECREATE your health and your life!

It gives us great pleasure to introduce you to the RECREATE 365 Journal. We are confident that this journal will make easy for you to learn and grow! ***Please focus on one chapter a week and complete all the assignments.***

We are going to coach you into a new lifestyle – not a diet – that you can embrace every day for the rest of your life. Go all in here, there will never be a time such as this so don't shortchange yourself! There is a lot of great information in this book and you will want to go back in from time to time and review it. Again, put your whole heart into your assignments. We believe in you! - Judy and Dr. Kobsar

4 Steps to Processing New Information

Here are the 4 levels of processing new information. This will help you understand the concept of 'waking up' and why this journal is going to be a tool for you to do so.

1. Unconscious Incompetence:

You don't know what you don't know. You are totally unaware, or in denial of certain situations existing in your life. People will try to explain, and you have no idea what they are talking about. You may even become defensive or irritated with them for bringing it up.

2. Conscious Incompetence:

You know that you don't know. You have an awareness of something, but no understanding of what exactly it is. You feel a pull inside of you. You have to do some research in order to move to the next level.

3. Conscious Competence:

You know that you know, and YOU ARE AWAKE! But you must think about and put into practice in order for growth to happen. Repetition rituals at the conscious competence level will shift your mind to unconscious competence.

4. Unconscious Competence:

You know, and you don't even have to think about it because it's become a reflex. It happens automatically.

The Teachability Index

How 'teachable' are you?
There are two variables of the teachability index.

First: What is your willingness to learn?

Rate yourself 1 to 10, with 10 being totally willing!

1   2   3   4   5   6   7   8   9   10

Second: What is your willingness to accept change?
What are you willing to give up in order to allow yourself to learn the lessons and make your dreams a reality?

Rate from 1 to 10

1   2   3   4   5   6   7   8   9   10

"When you change the way you look at things, the things you look at change."- Dr. Wayne Dyer.

How have you avoided using this wisdom in your life?

What excuses have you used to avoid making changes in your life?

List as many as you can and get really honest with yourself.
You may use the pages at the end of this book if you like.

Establishing Your Baseline and Goals with the Metabolic Assessment
Load your measurements into the BodySite app as outlined in your daily educational videos.

Your Metabolic Age at start of Recreate: _____ years old.

The Phase Angle test is like an EKG for your cells!
This test is the only way to measure the health of **ALL 70 trillion cells in your body.** It is vitally important to have a healthy heart, liver, and organs but it is next level to measure the health across the ENTIRE body population of cells.

Your Phase Angle = Your Cellular Health

Optimal	Average	Poor

Happy Cells, Happy Selves
The Phase Angle test measures the capacity of your cell membranes to hold an electrical charge. When your cells become unhealthy the membranes become unhealthy and can either become rigid and impermeable or they can begin to leak.

When the cell membrane is healthy and stable the higher the charge that it will be able to hold. Healthy cell membranes equate to healthy tissues and organs.

Factors that affect the Phase Angle are:
- Inflammation
- Chronic Disease
- Loss of Muscle
- Abusive Lifestyle
- Poor Nutrition
- Aging

BODY FAT PERCENT

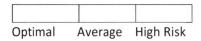

Optimal   Average   High Risk

	Optimal	**Average**	**High Risk**
Males	Below 15%	16 to 25%	Above 25%
Females	Below 20%	21 – 27%	Above 27%

HYDRATION

Optimal   Average   High Risk

	Optimal	**Average**	**High Risk**
Females	Above 60%	60 to 40%	Less than 40%
Males	Above 65%	65 to 40%	Less than 40%

BASAL METABOLIC RATE (BMR): _____

BMR: Total calories burned per day while at rest.

The quality of your calories is far more important than the quantity! However, to manage our weight effectively we must still consider the quantity of your total calories needed per day in addition to the quality of the food that you eat to achieve your health goals.

WEEK 1
The Birth of Quantum Physics

All Sickness and Disease Is Caused by an Energy Problem
Sickness and disease results from insufficient energy in the cells. Cells will shut down to conserve energy and the result is that oxygen and nutrients are unable to penetrate the cell wall which than starves the mitochondria (the powerhouse) of the cell.

- As your mitochondria go, so go your cells.
- As your cell goes, so goes your body.

Cells need oxygen, nutrients, and the ability to dispose of their waste. An energy shortage or an inability to dispose of waste will lead to cellular damage which becomes a disease. The type of disease is simply determined by the weakest link in your body systems.

The Birth of Quantum Physics: *the start of a science that proves the spiritual existence.*

In 1901 a brilliant scientist named Nikola Tesla wrote on his chalkboard:
- Human Energy = ½ Mass x Velocity^2

His formula surmised that one could increase their energy by having a spiritual practice like prayer or meditation, by eating clean food, exercising, or moving the body, and having meaningful relationships. In 1905 a guy with crazy white hair named Albert wrote on his chalkboard $E = MC^2$ and the world has never been the same since both of these discoveries.
- E = energy,
- MC^2 = everything else.

$E = MC^2$ is the most famous equation in the world – yet the world remains woefully and willfully unaware of the meaning and implications of Einstein's discovery in everyday life. One of the greatest illusions that still persists today is the idea that mass or matter is solid. Even a frying pan is ultimately a mass of vibrating energy. As we look into the pan, we find the iron atom, then the nucleus and ultimately, we have particles called 'quarks' which make up the protons and neutrons, and between the particles is space. However, the mass of the quarks is not enough to count for the heaviness of the pan – so where does that mass come from?

Energy does not just exist in matter, it is present in empty space – except that space is not empty, it is full of energy! That empty space full of energy manifests as 'virtual' particles that rapidly appear and disappear, and these particles give the fry pan its mass. Mass is just a way to carry energy as we see in trees, buildings, food, animals, and our bodies. Therefore, mass is just vibrating particles and space. Energy is the fundamental reality of the world we live in. Solid matter is a complete illusion.

Einstein himself said: "Concerning matter, we have been all wrong. What we called matter is energy, whose vibration has been so lowered as to be perceptible to the senses. There is no matter."

"Everything comes back to energy, especially your health."
Matter is just energy in a denser form or slower vibration and matter is just another form of the same fundamental nature of all of life – energy. Everything comes back to energy, especially your health. Health problems start with either a lack of energy or a destructive energy. Destructive energy was exploited by scientists like Oppenheimer in the 1930's who proved its effectiveness for making bombs however, it has been largely ignored when it comes to treating sickness and disease. 'Diagnosing' health conditions uses quantum

physics however, 'treating' them has been ignored for the most part. Using energy for treatment appears only where there are no effective drugs.

i.e. ultrasound is used to treat kidney stones.

Let's say that we knew a tumor was going to form in your liver in one week from now. For experimentation, we will do an MRI every day for 7 days. On day one, the MRI is clear, the same on days 2-6. On day 7 we begin to see abnormal cells in your kidney and do a biopsy.

Question: Where did the abnormal cells come from? The abnormal cells had to begin somewhere not physical. The abnormal cells came from energy. Before Einstein's discovery in 1905, we lived by the old standard of 'Newtonian physics' (Sir Isaac Newton and the apple) which told us atoms are solid matter.

We now know everything is energy and all energy has 3 common elements:

1. Frequency
2. Wavelength
3. Color spectrum

Some of the greatest scientific minds from all backgrounds including Nobel prize winners, recognize that the underlying cause of illness is always an energy issue.
- All living organisms emit an energy field. -Semyon Kirlian USSR
- The energy field starts it all. -Harold Burr PhD Yale University
- Body Chemistry is governed by quantum cellular fields. -Murray Gel-man PhD, Stanford University. Nobel Prize Laureate

The United States Department of Defense performed a study where they scraped the cells from the roof of a subject's mouth and placed them in a test tube hooked up to a lie detector. They also had the subject hooked to a lie detector but in a separate location in the same building and had him watch various programs on TV which had both violent and peaceful scenes. When watching the peaceful scenes on TV, the biology of both the subject and his cells calmed down. When watching stimulating programming, the subject and his cells showed arousal. They continued to separate the person and his cells up to 50 miles apart and for five days they still registered the same exact activity at the same exact time!

A similar experiment by Albert Einstein took two strangers and gave them a few minutes to get aquatinted and then separated them by 50 feet in a faraday (electromagnetic) cage to prevent radio frequency and other signals from going in or out. Then both individuals were hooked to an EEG and a pen light was shined into the eyes of the first subject (but not the other) causing pupil constriction, a normal response. Surprisingly, the pupil constriction occurred in both subjects at the same instant This explains the connection between a mother and her child and stories where a mom is having lunch in New York City and with a sudden horrified look says, "something happened to Jane, I must call my daughter". She immediately calls California to find out she was in an automobile accident but, she is OK.

MYSTICISM. Outside of the science of quantum physics these experiments may appear to be mystical but do we need to be afraid of Quantum Physics? No way! This is how the universe works and it's a fantastic breakthrough in health and healing.
- Copernicus discovered the earth and other planets revolve around the sun.
- Galileo proved Copernicus' theory with mathematics.

Both were persecuted for discovering scientific truths so don't expect to find a great understanding of quantum physics among the public or even from educators. I looked at my daughter's middle school science book and saw that they are still being taught the same old Newtonian physics I was taught 42 years ago. The tragedy is that we even knew back when I was in eighth grade, that this theory was outdated. It takes decades to change old mindsets especially when economic forces working against it. Fortunately, people are coming to understand the significance of quantum physics, in spite of it being ignored in our schools today. Scientists like Candace Pert PhD (discovered the adrenaline molecule in the 1970's), Caroline Leaf, PhD and Bruce Lipton PhD are modern day Galileo's and Copernicus' that are teaching and leading the charge in quantum physics.

Energy can take many forms!

Light energy encompasses a certain spectrum of frequency that is detected with our eyes. Sound frequencies are detected by our ears and bones. Infrared is felt as heat. There are many other frequencies of energy that we have no receptors in the body that are able to detect, which were one time thought to be mystical. X-rays, ultrasound, radar, etc... the list is infinite. There are three main components to frequencies:

1. **Frequency** changes from positive to negative in a certain time period. We call these cycles per second.

2. **Amplitude** is the magnitude of the wave above and below the baseline or zero point.

3. **Shape** of the wave, much like the different waves in the oceans, we can have a smooth sine wave, a spike wave, a square wave, etc.

What About Medicine and Frequency?

As mentioned earlier, using frequency for diagnosis is fairly common x-rays, EKGs, EEGs, MRI ... Frequency has been used in healing for decades in the back rooms of clinics. Royal Rife PhD was consistently treating cancer in the 1920s and 30s. Since his discoveries were a threat to the establishment he was discredited, and his lab and all his records mysteriously burned down. A similar story to Nikola Tesla's who was robbed of his patents for many discoveries including the radio and electricity patents that we still use today in homes, cell phones and laptops. Tesla was discredited for wanting to provide free and clean energy to all humanity but that threated the industrialists and dirty energy (oil, coal, etc.) In death, he was recognized and granted the patents as he was no longer a threat.

You Have to Have Power just like a car needs fuel and an oven needs electricity, you need food to function. The incredible thing about atomic energy is that its power was not created, it was released. The power that annihilated two cities in 1945 was always there in atoms. That same power lives in you and it can be constructive, lifting you to amazing heights and health or destructive, creating failure, disappointment and disease.

WEEK 2

30 Day Brain Surgery
How to Reprogram Your Brain

In 365 days, you will replace 98% of the cells in your body. It will happen automatically without any conscious effort on your part. How they turnover is massively affected by how you live your life however they will turn over either way. The remaining 2% is your brain and will only turn over by a conscious effort on your part. You can RECREATE your brain by learning to think in new ways.

Your conscious thinking will rewire your brain which will change your subconscious brain which operates 24 hours a day, 7 days a week. It determines how you react to circumstances in your life, how you treat others in your relationships and are the lenses of how you see the world.

Brain Programming:
Dr. John Sarno at New York University of medicine contends that chronic pain and disease are caused by repressed anger in the unconscious mind, rooted in our cell memories. These cellular memories are what drive your decisions every day. How you treat others, how you react to all situations and all of your emotions and it happens without you ever knowing it.

This is the SUBCONSCIOUS part of your brain. If we want to change our life, we must change our ASSOCIATIONS. Every single action you take has an effect on your destiny.

If we study destiny, we find everything in life has 4 parts:
1. Everything we think or do is a cause set in motion.
2. Every thought and action has an effect or result in our life.

3. Our results "stack up" to take our lives in a particular direction.
4. For every direction there is an ultimate destination or destiny.

3 KEYS WE HAVE LEARNED UP TO THIS POINT

Key #1 <u>Stress is the source of most health issues.</u>
Healing the source of the problem is proven by a technology called Heart Rate Variability (HRV).

Key #2 <u>Every problem is an energy problem.</u>
When you heal the energy, you can heal the problem.

Key #3 <u>Issues of the heart (cell memories) are the healing mechanisms for health.</u>
Cellular memories can resonate destructive energy frequencies that create illness. Heal the heart and you heal many problems.

Emotional issues always take a backseat to healing, why?

1. No one wants to admit they have them
2. If they do, they don't want to talk about them
3. We don't effectively treat them with conventional health care.

According to Stanford University researcher Dr. Bruce Lipton, false beliefs are embedded in cell memories. If you don't heal cellular memories from life traumas you will have bad programming that signal cells to cause disease. For years, scientists believed that memories were stored in the brain. To determine where in the brain, they cut out just about every part of it only to find the memories remained largely intact. Though memories can be stimulated from certain areas of the brain - the actual storage does not appear confined to the brain. So, where are they stored? The answer first appeared with organ transplants. People started having the thoughts, feelings, food cravings of the organ donor. Today many scientists are convinced that memories are stored in cells all over the body. Southwestern University medical school published a study in September 2004 which reported that healing mechanisms in the body may be in the cellular memories. They found that as the cell memories of the organism go, so goes the health of the organism.

"Treating Humans without energy is treating dead matter."
-Albert Gyorgi MD, Nobel Prize Laureate

The institute of Heart Math performed research that placed human DNA in a test tube and instructed the subjects of that DNA to think painful thoughts or destructive memories. The DNA was literally damaged. Next, they put the same DNA back in the test tube and instructed them to think positive, happy memories which healed the DNA.

Why positive thinking doesn't heal cellular memories
Mechanisms in the subconscious mind shelter destructive memories from being healed. When you successfully heal memories, you no longer think the negative beliefs or feel the negative emotions of anger, frustration, resentment, guilt, hopelessness, etc.

Coping Is Not Healing.
Most counseling therapy, and self - help programs provide 'coping mechanisms' which are helpful and often necessary in the short term just like a medication for heart or liver disease. The medication (or counseling) helps the problem, but we can't just stop there if we want to truly heal the root cause and restore our health! Coping does not address the underlying cause of the problem. The coping allows you to be productive in life but does not resolve the root cause of the issue.

"Coping allowed me to turn my life around. I completed my doctorate, found, and married the woman of my dreams, created the Wellness Method, ran a successful practice and have a wonderful family. So, I do not want to minimize the benefits of coping but coping makes you numb inside. You cannot truly feel the wonders that life has to offer because coping teaches how to "manage" your pain. Unfortunately, it also inhibits the full experience of positive feelings in life. Only, true healing allows you to feel emotions again." – Dr. Brad Kobsar

CHANGE YOUR ASSOCIATIONS AND THOUGHTS to serve you.
There are three steps to RECREATE your brain in 30 days, with each phase cut into 10-day increments.

PHASE 1
10 DAY BRAIN DETOXIFICATIONS:

Eliminate "Stinkin Thinkin", which are associations and thoughts that limit you in life and replace them with new thoughts that set you up for success.

Your Assignment:
In the blank pages at the back of this journal, write down IN PENCIL OR BLUE PEN every limiting belief, every repetitive negative thought, that you encounter about yourself in the following categories:

- Spiritual
- Intellectual
- Emotional
- Physical
- Relationships
- Finances
- Professional

Leave a space of 3 or 4 lines right after each limiting belief.

3 Examples

1. Physical: I am not ____enough (fit, good looking, old/young, etc.)

2. Intellectual: I'm not _____enough (smart, have a degree in, etc.)

3. Financial:
   - Money is the root of all evil.
   - I was born poor
   - Money is not important.

4. Professional:
   - I do not have connections.
   - I am not an entrepreneur.
   - It is too much work.
   - I will not have enough time for my family, etc.

Get all these negative beliefs on paper. It might not feel great but we must recognize them so we can demolish them.

PHASE 2
10 DAYS TO PLANT NEW SEEDS AND GROW NEW THOUGHTS

You have to perform mental repetitions just like exercising your muscles at the gym so new healthy thoughts are automatic.

Your Assignment:
a) Write down a NEW BELIEF under each LIMITING BELIEF that overrides the limiting belief … like noise cancelling headphones! These beliefs will serve you; they are full of hope and positive words.

b) Write them in RED INK. Go through all of your limiting beliefs and write a new belief under it in red. Even if you don't 'believe' that new belief, write it anyway.

2 Examples:

1. Financial:
   - Money is the root of all evil. -Old limiting belief
   - The love of money is the root of all evil, in my hand's money will do good in the world because I am a good person.   -New Belief

2. Professional:
   - I'm not old / young / smart / fit / rich enough to get the job done/ finish the project/start the business. -Old limiting belief
   - I am old enough to have the experience to make wise decisions. I am young enough to have the time and energy to accomplish my goals. - New Beliefs

For each of the actions you listed above: Write down 3 reasons why you must change that behavior now; and list the reasons you can do it.

PHASE 3
10 DAYS TO AUTOMATIZE NEW THOUGHTS and **ACT ON THEM.**

I. Now that you have 'limiting beliefs' and 'new beliefs written out in all categories, for the next 7-14 days read them both through all of your pages. Soon you will automatically want to only read the new beliefs written it red. They will feel better day by day as you read through them.

II. When you read the new beliefs, <u>you must believe them in your heart, or the exercise will not work.</u> If you do not believe your new beliefs, keep reading them daily until you do. Thinking about change is not enough. You have to implement the new thoughts into your life so that they become part of your cellular make up.

III. After about 2 weeks or so you will feel like it is time to erase those old thoughts written in blue. Go ahead and SCRATCH THEM OUT with black pen so you can no longer see them.

IV. Continue reading your new beliefs daily for another 2 weeks. Meditate on your new beliefs until they become the automatic go to.

V. Take the next 21 days to walk out the new thoughts and beliefs so they become who you are and program it into your cell memory.

CONGRATULATIONS! YOU COMPLETED THE BRAIN DETOX!

Interrupting the signal

The brain is the control center. It detects and sends energy frequencies through your nervous system, telling all body systems what to do. The hypothalamus in the brain sends emergency signals to the body when a threat is present. When there is no real emergency and we go into fight or flight mode, the frequencies are destructive in the form of chronic disease. Healing changes destructive energy signals into healthy ones. The way to do this is relatively simple.

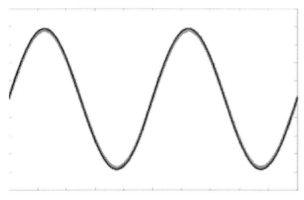

Here is a sine wave: Assume that this is the energy frequency of cancer.

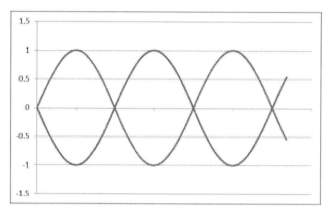

The way to the change that frequency is to hit it with one that is exactly opposite, it would look like this.

The Physics of Noise Canceling Headphones

Noise canceling headsets block out background noise. When you turn on the switch a microphone records the outside noise and creates an exact opposite frequency to the noise and cancels it out. This is the quantum physics of healing in a nutshell.

A healing frequency stops the hypothalamus from sending that 911 signal when it is sent in error. Heart Rate Variability (HRV) is the gold standard for measuring stress in the Autonomic Nervous System which combines the sympathetic (fight or flight) and parasympathetic (calming) nervous system.

Change the Frequency Heal the Problem

WEEK 3

Change Your Thoughts, Change Your World

It's imperative to begin to think about and answer these 2 questions

1. What is your ultimate purpose in life?

2. What do you want your life to be about?

While few people know precisely how their lives will turn out, we can decide in advance the kind of person we want to become and how we want to live our lives. Having this "bigger purpose" can pull us through some of the short term, tough times and keep things in perspective, allowing us to remain happy fulfilled and driven to achieve our dreams.

What do you presently create in your world?

Do you create joy? Stress? Frustration?

What kinds of feelings do you create in your spouse/partner?

What do you create in your family?

What do you create in your work? your community, your city, etc?

How do you create it?

CHESTERTON'S 5 STAGES OF CHANGE:
If you see some things that you do not like and would like to change them, take a moment to consider where you are in the change process.

1. Pre-contemplation stage
This is when we don't even know that something needs to change. You think your mindset is fine, you may be in denial or you may feel unrest in your heart. Do you feel unrest?

Do you desire more from life?

2. Contemplation stage
You begin to consider change, but barriers arise from 'Stinkin Thinkin'.

Excuses and blame- If you are in the habit of blaming others (parents, family, etc) for the things in your life, this needs to be addressed. Wellness begins with self - responsibility.

"It's too late to change." Delete this thought! Your brain can be re-wired, no matter your age.

"I'll do it later"-Procrastination is the killer of dreams! Do not let this once in a lifetime opportunity pass you by. You have the science and the support to RECREATE your life. Now is the time!

"I can't do this." This is negative self-talk that many struggle with and don't even realize it. Imagine programming positive, beautiful thoughts all day long… how would that feel? Demolish 'can't'.

Note: You started this new process in the 30 - day Brain Detox.

3. Preparation stage
You are ready, you have a plan and a system in RECREATE 365!

4. Action stage
Commit to the exercises in your journal, this is you taking action.

5. Mastery
Change becomes permanent and in Wellness Mastery you have the practices, skills, and tools to live in that zone. What's most important, you will get education all throughout your Recreate program so that if you veer off track, you will know how to get back on!

Mind Gym
Exercise Your Brain, Change Your Life!

Now that YOU have decided to change your life, let's get clear on all your goals in all areas of your life!

Just like training to improve your physical skills in sports like football, tennis, basketball, soccer, or hockey – in order to be a well-balanced, all - around athlete you need cross training. In your Mind Gym, you will use a three-prong approach to training that starts with goal setting that is followed by an accountability structure that you will use to submit to. This is what will bring you the discipline needed to achieve your goals. You completed the first part of goal setting in the previous weeks, now let's get more detailed!

1. **SPARKLE**: This is the first step - set goals for all areas of your life.
2. **Daily CRUSH**: 10 minutes every day to set yourself up to crush your goals and crush the day.
3. **Triggers and Rituals:** New actions every day to change your life.

What's the difference between winners and losers? ONE MORE STEP
You can't always win, that's just life. However, the way you react in life is what separates people and determines your level of success and especially your happiness. Now it's your turn to dream.

Answer these questions:
1. What would you attempt to do if you knew you could not fail?

2. How do you want to grow?

3. What areas of your life need work?

- What do you need to get better organized in your personal life or your professional life?

- What do you need to Learn or to study to set me on the right path for my life?

- What Fear(s) do you need to Overcome that are stopping you from really going for it in your life?

- Who do you want more quality time with and to deepen your relationship with?

If you are like most people, you would shoot for the moon! You would set your sights SKY high because after all, what do you have to lose?

Many people might answer this question with, "What if I fail?" Fear of failure is real, so I want to share with you a couple of **secrets** from successful people.

Turn a Bad Day into Good Data. You can learn a lot about success when you study how successful people 'fail' and apply those lessons to their tomorrow.
Successful people 'fail' more times than the average person even attempts to try something. Nikola Tesla made thousands of unsuccessful attempts at inventing electricity and when asked,

> *"Isn't it a shame that with the tremendous amount of work you have done you haven't been able to get any results?"*

Tesla turned like a flash, and with a smile replied,

> *"Results! Why man, I have gotten lots of results! I know several thousand things that won't work!"*

To eliminate fear and doubt, we must change our thoughts about them. First, define what must happen for you to feel successful and to feel like a failure, then create new definitions for what must happen for you to feel success or failure.

Definition of Failure:

Definition of Success:

What Would Make Your Life SPARKLE?!

What do you want to create in your life? If you had no restrictions and were guaranteed success, what would your life look like? Here are the 6 areas of life that will make you SPARKLE.

Spiritual	Your alignment with your authentic self and with God, The Creator, The Divine energy, whichever name you prefer. What matters is that you are aligned. This is the foundation that life is built upon.
Physical	<ul><li>Your cells, tissues, organs, etc.</li><li>Your metabolism and hormones.</li><li>Your diet and nutrition.</li></ul>
Attitude= Altitude ie: how high you will soar in life.	All events are neutral. They are not positive or negative. YOU assign the meaning to them. The short time between an event and the interpretation we make in our brain is determined by your Attitude. It directs the path you set for your entire life. The meanings you assign to events in life are from your lenses of the world which result from your experiences, faith, and belief.
Relationships	Family, friends, co-workers, etc.
Knowledge	What do you need to learn for the life you want? Certifications, degrees, internships, etc.
Livelihood	The amount of money you need or want to earn. Tax strategies, financial planning, etc.
Educator	Sharing your bright light with the world is why we are here. The more we grow & develop ourselves, the more we have to share. Teaching forces you to really own a subject so the best way to really learn is to teach it. What can you teach to help others?

ASSIGNMENT:

Rank each of the categories of your life in SPARKLE, from 1 to 10.
10 being the Best and 1 being the worst

By completing this assignment, it will help you to see where you need to focus more of your time and energy.

RANKING 1 to 10

S _____

P _____

A _____

R _____

K _____

L _____

E _____

Week 4
What is your WHY – Coaching Call

Each week you will focus on one section of your journal. If you don't finish a section, go at your own pace. This is meant to guide you in phases through your mindset work. In this section you will be clearly defining your goals for your Recreate Program and you will be discovering your motivation behind your desire to improve your health.

The Learning Balance Scale: Two Sides of the scale.

Thinking Side: Lives in the mind. The following words are associated with this side: thoughts, thinking, desires, dreams, goals, attitude, mental processes, objectives, vibration, intention, energy, motivation, and emotions.

Action Side: Involves actions. The following are associated with this side: physical movements, techniques, strategies, action steps and activities.

Thought = the Why, Action = the How.
In theory there should be a balance of both, but the thinking scale is 99% more important than the action scale. Reflect and rate your place on the Training Balance Scale of 1 to 10:

Reflect on where you are on this scale. Be honest with yourself. If you think and talk about your goals and dreams all the time, but you have not made much progress in the last few years, then you are going to rate more on the thinking side (1-5). If you think about your goals and get moving, even if you are failing, you are still DOING! You are going to rate more on the Action side (5-10).

Rate yourself again here:

1 = Thinking Side   10 = Action Side

1   2   3   4   5   6   7   8   9   10

COACHING CALL

When you know what your goals are and are clear on YOUR WHY, you will succeed!

1) Write down your general overall health goals.

1.

2.

3.

"Motivation gets you started; Results keep you going."
Fail Forward: Set up your life so it's impossible to fail. Here's a great view on 'failure' that we want you to adopt. Successful people decide the only way to fail is to GIVE UP AND QUIT. So, for them, there is no such thing as failure, only different results from continuously trying. Look, we all trip up - you won't hit a home run every time you step up to bat. In fact, you will miss more often than not- but you can either quit or you can 'FAIL FORWARD' and keep moving.

Your WHY is your foundation and motivation for change and it will be something you will go back to again and again as you move through your Recreate Program. It will be the "wind beneath your wings".

Your Why drives your success!

2) WHY #1 What **H**urts **Y**ou if you don't follow through?

What happens to the people in your life if you fail at your goals? List all the regrets you will have to face if you don't succeed in this journey to restore your health:

3) WHY #2 What **H**elps **Y**ou … if you do follow through?

List all that you will gain. What happens to the people in your life if you achieve your goals? All the ways your life will change for the better when you reach your health goals:

4) A year from now, when you have reached your health goals and are setting new ones, what will you be saying to yourself and what will you be doing?

Phrase your answers in these terms.

*- **I am** hiking often and moving well!*

5) What are the potential barriers that could get in the way of you reaching your goals and being that person, you just described.

Your Assignment:

WEEK 5
CREATE A LIFE THAT WILL SPARKLE

Goals Create Your Destiny, they compel you to succeed in life and give you purpose to drive you forward. Who you become in the process of achieving your goals is far more important than the results! Make your goals inspiring!! List your goals in each facet of SPARKLE. Dare to dream and do not over analyze... just write!

___30___ Days _____ months _____ years	**S**piritual I will read a daily passage from a book about spiritual growth
_____ Days ___6___ Months _____ Years	**P**hysical I will lose 40 pounds
_____ Days _____ Months ___2___ Years	**A**ttitude Repair my relationship with my daughter.
_____ Days _____ Months _____ Years	**R**elationships
_____ Days _____ Months _____ Years	**K**nowledge (certifications, degrees, etc.)
_____ Days _____ Months _____ Years	**L**ivelihood
_____ Days _____ Months _____ Years	**E**ducator

What would you have to believe to consistently follow through on your life transformation?

Part of what drives us in life is our desire. Seeing and admitting that things are not as good as we want them to be creates a drive to make our lives the way we believe they should and must be.

Your Assignment:
1. Write 1 decision you've been putting off or that if you make them now, will change your life in each category of SPARKLE?

S

_____

P

_____

A

_____

R

_____

K

_____

L

_____

E

_____

2. Set a timeline for each of the goals you set for yourself in the box with the blank space for days, months and years. Fill in the time that you are committed to accomplishing it. i.e., 1-5 month, years.

3. Write 1 action you can take today toward to change your life in each category of SPARKLE?

S

_____

P

_____

A

_____

R

_____

K

_____

L

_____

E

_____

4. The rocking chair test, created by Anthony Robbins can help you achieve your goals. Imagine yourself much older, sitting in your chair, looking back on your life, first, as if you had not successfully achieved your goals then imagine yourself having achieved them.

WEEK 6

Morning MAGIC – Daily CRUSH – Evening MAGIC

Congratulations! You are on your way to successfully reprogramming your brain!

Let's move forward into the next phase and begin to make your life Magical!

MORNING MAGIC: The 5 Minute Power Morning
For your new thoughts to become 'automatic' you must practice and develop the skills to overcome your old habits. Here you will find exercises to begin re-wiring your brain so that your thoughts work IN your favor and so you can begin designing the thought-life that you desire!

First Minute, let's say you begin at 9am

Power Exercise
Start each day thinking of 1 thing and 1 person you are grateful for in your life right now. Say out loud or in your head why you are grateful, imagine in your mind connecting with them, feeling the emotion of gratefulness. You brain cannot feel sadness or anger while you are feeling grateful, so you must fully embrace the feeling of gratefulness. It can be big or small.

- I am grateful for my life, so I wake up every day expecting something powerful to happen.
- I am grateful for my brain and the freedom to choose my thoughts to create my life.
- I am grateful for my spouse, my children who enrich my life every day.

Minute 2, 9:02am
SPARKLE

Pull out your path to make your life SPARKLE - remind yourself of your unlimited potential and your most important priorities. Read them out loud from top to bottom. As you focus on what's most important to you, your level of internal motivation will increase Reading your commitments, your purpose, and what your goals are, re-energizes you to take the actions necessary to live the life you truly want, deserve, and now know is possible for you. *Take notes if you like*

Minute 3, 9:03am
Acknowledge WHO you are.

Read over the reminders of how capable you *really* are and the gifts you have been blessed with.

MINUTE 4, 9:04am
Align your heart with your purpose in the world.

Remember that your purpose gives you a feeling of confidence!

MINUTE 5, 9:05am
Visualization

Close your eyes, or look at your vision board, or dream journal and visualize your goals. What will it look and feel like when you reach them? Visualize the day going perfectly and see yourself enjoying your work, smiling, and laughing with your family, your significant other, and easily accomplishing all that you intend to accomplish for that day. Imagine what it will look like and feel like and experience the joy of what you will create.

Minutes 6 – 15
Daily CRUSH

10 Minutes to crushing your goals. The seemingly, small actions that you take each day once you master these skills will build the foundation to create the life you desire. Once you decide how you want to live, you can create the mindset that supports it.

In the Daily CRUSH exercise, you will begin reading an inspirational book daily and follow the instructions in the table below.

Here are some spiritual and inspirational books that we recommend using during your Daily Crush exercises:

- The Biology of Belief -Dr. Bruce H. Lipton, PhD
- Switch on Your Brain -Dr. Caroline Leaf
- The Molecules of Emotion -Candace Pert PhD
- The Science of being Great -Wallace Wattles
- See You at the Top -Zig Ziglar
- The Field -Lynn McTaggart
- Awaken the Giant -Anthony Robbins
- How to Win Friends and Influence People -Dale Carnegie
- Think and Grow Rich -Napoleon Hill
- The Healing Code -Lloyd and Johnson
- Change Your Thoughts, Change Your Life -Dr. Wayne Dyer
- The Bible - the 'original' personal development book -God

Daily Crush
Do this Daily CRUSH Exercise for the next 21 days and we encourage you to continue this for the rest of your life!

**Use the CRUSH templates in the back of this journal.

Capture: Read a paragraph, verse, or small section	Read a paragraph, verse, or section from a book of your choice. **Capture** a passage that gets your attention. Something positive, uplifting, or inspiring. When we **"capture,"** the amygdala in our brain provides input to the mind about the emotions connected to the thoughts.
Reflect: Focus on the small section and write it down.	Find 3 - 5 words the passage you captured that really stood out. When we **"reflect"** the thalamus and hypothalamus provide motivation.
Unite: Write the 3 - 5 words to activate the brain.	Write the 3-5 words down three times. When we **"write,"** the central hub in our brains consolidate our thoughts. MRI's show increased neural activity in sections of the brain to sharpen the gray matter, to activate "positive" thoughts, healing, and memory.
Silence: Take 5 minutes to go inside and write your observations.	Ask yourself and the Creator, God, **"What do you want me to hear?"** Be silent and meditate on the phrase. The heart is a checking station to help us hear healthy thoughts to replace old toxic ones. Record in your journal what you have **'heard'**. Use the blank pages in the back of your journal for this exercise
Healthy Acts: Implement this message in my life today?	Use whatever you learned from this exercise in your life today. This is where we practice using new healthy thoughts until it becomes automatic. This is where your words and actions line up with new beliefs and emotions. This happens in the limbic system and helps your mind-heart congruence occurs. By using the new thought at least 2 times today, we can ingrain it forever.

Rituals take on many shapes and forms, sometimes in community or in solitude. People have rituals for many reasons, reducing stress, boosting confidence and even competition.

- Michael Jordan wore his North Carolina shorts underneath his Chicago Bulls shorts in every game.

- Curtis Martin, of the New York Jets reads Psalms 91 before every game.

- Anthony Robbins has a ritual called "Priming," in three-parts:

  1. 3 sets of 30 Kapalbhati Pranayama breaths.
  2. Closes eyes, slows breathing, express gratitude.
  3. Prays for help, guidance, and strength thru the day.

- Steve Jobs founder of Apple computers made his bed, showered, and then look in the mirror in his eyes and asked,

  "If today was the last day of my life, would I be happy with what I'm about to do today?"

If the answer was "no" too many days in a row, he made a change.

EVENING MAGIC: 5 Minute PM Power Evening: end the day with these simple but powerful tools:

*Keep a bedside journal to record any thoughts that arise in this process.

The first 3 minutes can be done alone or if you prefer, share with your spouse or family to bring you closer together. When sharing with others, dinner or bedtime are good options.

MINUTE 1: List 1 amazing thing that happened today.

MINUTE 2: What could I have done to make today better?

MINUTE 3: How can I be 1% better tomorrow? [SEP]

MINUTE 4: Align with God your creator! Take time to remember that you are connected to the Almighty and He gave you life, blessings and a purpose to fulfill in this world.

MINUTE 5: Align with your purpose in this world. Acknowledge your purpose and you will gain confidence to push ahead. Know that you are doing what you were created for and are using the gifts that you were blessed with by the creator.

WHO AM I?

I Am your constant companion.
I am your greatest helper or your heaviest burden.
I will push you onward or drag you down to failure.
I am completely at your command.

Half the things you do, you might just as well turn over to me,
and I will be able to do them quickly and correctly.
I am easily managed; you must merely be firm with me.
Show me exactly how you want something done, and after a few
lessons I will do it automatically.

I am the servant of all great men.
And, alas, of all failures as well.
Those who are great, I have made great.
Those who are failures, I have made failures.

I am not a machine, though I work with all the precision of a machine.
Plus, the intelligence of a man.
You may run me for profit, or run me for ruin; it makes no difference to
me.

Train me, be firm with me and I will put the world at your feet.
Be easy with me, and I will destroy you.
Who am I?

I am Your HABIT!

WEEK 7
Cellular Memories

The Power of Belief
The power of belief is also known as the **placebo effect** and the **nocebo effect**. What is so interesting about quantum physics is that it changes reality by the way we look at it. Or as Dr. Wayne Dyer so brilliantly stated, "When you change the way you look at things, the things you look at change."

You may have an **Anti-Virus Program** on your computer but guess what, you have a similar program on your conscious and unconscious mind called your heart and soul. Within our human hard drive is a stimulus response program. It is basically an instinct to **seek pleasure** and **avoid pain**. When children cannot use logic, they operate on a more pain pleasure principle. We know as adults that a child's reactions are not necessarily logical. A child may find pleasure in eating ice cream until they are sick or may be so scared and worried about a spider that they cannot even enjoy life.

3 Types of Memories We Often Can't Recall:
These memories become a stimulus-response, a protective programming belief system.

1.Inherited memories
We all inherit DNA memories from our parents that are stored in our cells. Cellular memories can be good and bad, and they can be healed. It is impossible to address problems that you don't know exist, but fortunately there are tests to find them.

2.Pre-language and pre-logical thinking memories
Before we were able to think rationally or articulate very well, we had many events occur in our life and they are interpreted through the reasoning filters at the time of the experience. In the first six years of

life we live in a 'delta theta' brainwave state which means our experiences are hardwired without a logical filter we develop as we mature If a baby wakes at 2am with wet diapers they cry out to eliminate their discomfort. If the mother wakes and is rough or upset, the baby will want to avoid being mistreated and will not understand how hard the mom works or how tired she is. They only know that if they have one pain, they will experience another (angry parent). They also feel the right to be clean, dry, and cared for and this confusion gets stored as a pre-language memory that may be triggered every time, they should ask to have a physical need met.

3. Trauma Memories

If a person graduates with honors from a top school and is nominated for greatness but falls short, they may self-sabotage, and think "Everyone says I should be a force in life, but every time I get close, I mess it up" This thinking can revert to a day when a sibling got a popsicle for finishing lunch while she did not. The 5-year-old was in Delta -Theta brain state. A phenomenon of trauma memories is that your rational brain disconnects because it goes into a degree of shock similar to a parent's brain when their child is in danger.

A 5-year-old reasons ... "mom gave sissy a popsicle but not me which means she loves her more. There's something wrong with me so other people won't love me either." This feeling becomes deeply ingrained and a self-fulfilling prophecy, so they often struggle in life until the memory is healed.

The Stress Response- When the Unconscious Mind Takes Over. Stanford University researcher Dr. Bruce Lipton talks about people who are afraid that shouldn't be. These memories - inherited; pre-language; pre-logical; trauma - are a stimulus response, belief system. A protective system where pain memories are given priority so that when reactivated we re-experience them and our logical thinking is diminished.

When something in our present occurs that is associated with a past trauma, it is reactivated in the unconscious. A great secret that few people know is that when you do things you don't want to, think things you don't want to, feel things you don't want to -you have a reactivated memory.

The Heart Knows Only the Present
When a past memory is reactivated from 20 years ago, it's experienced again, right now. There is no rhyme or reason for this state of confusion and conflict, but it feels extraordinarily strong and demands attention. We try to rationalize it by using self-help approaches to find an explanation to the blocks we experience. Your protective programming is a deeply encoded belief system based on memories so by the time you get to 6, 8 or 10 years old you have ingrained memories for many things - relationships, identity, success, a good person, a worthy person and so on.

Logical mind is Bypassed.
The intensity of the painful event, the more stress hormones are released and the wider the perception of what is defined as a similar situation years later. The bigger the trauma, the more reactivation and over - reaction years later of the program which can make people sick. Your unconscious mind protects trauma memories from healing because it interprets that as unsafe since the memories protect the person from pain.

So, how to heal trauma memories? People spend thousands of dollars and decades of life trying to overcome the wrong programming to liberate the life they desire. However, this will not happen by using 'will power' to change. You must address the source – the issues of the heart.

LACK OF BELIEF

As your brain develops, another belief system is formed with language and logic, based on the stimulus response belief system. Since 1886, runners tried and failed, to break the 4-minute mile. Roger Bannister broke through 10 Years after a group of medical researchers 'proved' the 4-minute barrier could not be done. In 1954 Bannister broke the 4-minute mark and 46 days Later, John Landy did it and a year later, 3 runners broke the barrier in a single race.

What are the 4 - minute miles in your life? Are they because of UNBELIEF? If you can believe the truth, the mental blocks will fall away. 90% of our beliefs are subconscious so our rational beliefs are built upon the stimulus response protective belief system. So, when you say "I believe", you are saying it consciously but not subconsciously.

All Destructive Habits are rooted in HEART memories. To truly heal them, not just cope, you must heal the source. Mental health experts know that women with eating disorders believe something untrue. Many beautiful women can look in a mirror and see something different. This is a clear case of destructive heart pictures and stress response beliefs. What most don't understand is that this phenomenon happens on a continuum from totally deception to 100% truth. Take the field of sports and peak performance. Star athletes: Steph Curry, Sidney Crosby, Roger Federer, etc.... visualize their game because at the professional level, 90% of the game is mental.

YOUR BELIEFS CAN HEAL YOU OR HURT YOU

Researchers at Stanford University found that the trigger for disease is always a false belief and once we believe the truth, we become impervious to disease. If your beliefs are loving and truthful you will develop exceptional abilities in whatever you do.

Finding hidden beliefs- How do you know if you are having a stimulus response belief?

1. **Feelings:** if they don't match your current circumstances, you are likely stuck in a stimulus response pain memory reactivation so, ask a friend, "This is my situation and here's how I'm feeling. Please be honest with me, is this sensible?"
2. **Thoughts:** Pain memories means your living in the past.
3. **Behaviors:** repeating things you don't want and that work against you is acting on a pain memory.
4. **Loss of conscious control** Coping is the popular way to deal with problems but, it treats symptom not the underlying
5. **Healing the heart is the only way to resolve pain!**

When the heart and head conflict, the heart always wins
'Pictures' not 'words' are the language of the heart! Imagination is the picture maker! People who have lost the ability to imagine usually have more pain memories.

"Guard your heart above all else because from it flows the issues of life." - Proverbs 4:23

Stanford University researcher Bruce Lipton states that it's nearly impossible to change our issues through will power because the subconscious is 1 million times stronger than willpower.

1. **You are who you are in your heart**.
You may tell people this is who I am, this is what I believe this is what I've done ... but who you are in your heart always wins.

2. **You are where you are based on what's in your heart.**
   The stimulus response belief system, when activated, will take you back to the age you were when that pain memory was created.

3. **You Do What You Do**
   Based on what is in your heart

4. **The heart is programmed to protect**
   Your priorities are determined by what's in your heart. The only way to live and love from the heart in the way we want to, is to heal the destructive memories of the heart.

Confusion Blocks Truth
You need to heal destructive heart memories which cause you to believe lies. Confusion is caused by 3 things:

1. **Cell memories** that conflict with each other.
2. **Conflict** between the conscious and unconscious mind.
3. **Illogical Thinking:** emotions from the memories compromises rational reasoning.

The Peace Test: is the litmus test for this confusion
1. **It is Peace, Anxiety or Numbness?**
   True peace is not situation dependent it is faith dependent. If your faith is weak, you will be tossed like waves in the sea with every storm that comes your way.
2. **Numbness.**
   No anxiety, no fear, no pain ... BUT you feel nothing! This is a result of so much past destruction that your heart memory turned off your feeler to help you survive the pain.

The Missing Ingredients
1. Clarify your goals - results you want.
2. Power to achieve the results.
3. BELIEF releases Power! You must Believe the truth to get the sustained results we desire.

30 Years Ago, ADD and ADHD Didn't Exist. Mental illness has exploded, and the root cause is destructive memories. TV and movies are filled with deceit, sex, murder... (and don't even get me started on all the drug and fast-food commercials) all of which go into our cellular memories which block your success and make you sick. Dr. Bruce Lipton showed that 100% of stress that makes us sick is wrong beliefs. Destructive memories have some truth but what is false is our interpretations.

- I am worthless,
- I'm never safe,
- No one will ever look at me the same way.

It may seem like a daunting task to have to find a whole truth before you can have a sustain results but don't despair, it's not that hard. If we have a relatively clean heart, we will know the truth when we see or hear it. It resonates and we feel it in our core. However, when there are too many lies in the heart, the conscience is drowned out or confused by competing voices. What heals the issues of the heart is replacing lies with the truth. Healing through prayer resolves the underlying cause not just coping strategy mentioned earlier. If you have a career, relationship or financial issue in your life rest assured that you are blocking your breakthrough with a misunderstanding of the truth. **Belief and Truth is always at the root of health problems.**

What Is Healing

Our wellness partners struggle with problems ranging from disease, mental illness, obesity, relationship struggles, addictions. We always ask two questions:
1.what should you be doing differently in relation to your problem?

2. why aren't you doing it?

We have a multi - million-dollar book industry with techniques and programs that don't work for people who desperately need help? Answer: NONE of those things heal the source of the problem.

Miracles or Just A New Paradigm
God built the possibility of miraculous healing into us as part of his original intention for the world, and it is still available to us today.
The Mechanism
Research From the institute of heart math identified an internal healing resource so powerful it literally has a healing effect on damaged DNA.

Prayer is always the first course of action.
Words are important but they are just a tool like a hammer. What's most important is your relationship with you and the Creator and it has to come from your heart.

Prayer Puts Healing on Steroids
But you have to find out where you are wounded so that you know what to pray for. We will cover the what in the next chapter but let's give you one step in the "HOW to pray."

The Prayer for Healing
- From the book, the Healing Code by Dr. Alex Lloyd.

Think of any heart issues you are aware of and identify the emotion you feel. Rate all issues from 1 to 10, see if any cell memories come up and rate that memory in terms of how much it bothers you. Rate the memory. Work on early or strongest memory until it's below a one then move on until they're all down to zero or one. Insert any issues you are aware of in the blank space.

You will uncover more issues from the assessment in the next chapter but for now start using this prayer for those already know about.

"I pray that all known and unknown negative images, unhealthy beliefs, destructive cellular memories, and all physical issues related to your problem or issues of …….

…. would be found, opened and healed by filling me with the light, life and love of God. Pray that the effectiveness of this healing be increased by 100 times or more - Telling the body to make healing a priority.

WEEK 8

Heart Healing - Coaching Call

The Heart Issues Finder:
This is designed by Dr. Alex Lloyd, the author of the Healing Code. He created this assessment which is a powerful tool to uncover cell memories that you may be unaware of. Healing begins by identifying the issues which can take thousands of dollars and years of therapy. I am not saying that this can replace therapy completely however, it's a great start to revealing some past memories that we were too young to even be aware of.

The Free Assessment and Personalized Report of your heart problems can be found at this link:
https://www.thehealingcodes.com/newhif/en/assessment/process.php
Take the assessment to learn where you have some healing issues.

12 CATEGORIES.

3 Inhibitor Categories
Designed to remove garbage from our lives -- DETOX

1. Unforgiveness
The most critical. In the Lord's prayer it is the only issue that Jesus addresses twice. Unforgiveness is often anger or irritation or not wanting to be around a certain person. Forgiveness is enlightened self - interest.

2. Harmful Actions
weight issues diet, exercise, addictions, etc. .... all are heart issues.
- They all fall into either one of two categories:
  - i. self - protection   or   ii. self - gratification

3. Wrong Beliefs

9 Core Healing Categories

- Designed to instill the seeds that will grow in life, health, and prosperity. A healthy home is not just free of garbage, it permeates joy, peace for a resting and caring place that transforms the hearts who live there or visit.
- Each category has a virtue that needs to be instilled and a destructive opposite to demolish. There is one body system in each core category.

4. Love Vs Selfishness; love means putting yourself aside and choosing pain. Sex is not making love; it is a celebration of love. The body system for love is the endocrine system. So, if you are low, your hormones are affected.

5. Joy Vs Sadness: Joy is the most faked emotion. We are taught to put on a happy face. The body system is the skin. Sadness is the lie of hopelessness.

6. Peace Vs Anxiety /Fear: Endocrine and hormones.

7. Patience Vs Anger/Frustration/Impatience: indicator of comparing self to others leading to inferiority or superiority. An unhealthy feeling that something has to change for me to be okay. Body system is the immune system. The most direct way to heal is RAK's.

8. **Kindness Vs Rejection\Harshness;** harsh with people out of their own pain and feelings of rejection. Body system is the CNS (brain & spinal cord).

9. **Goodness Vs Not Being Good Enough:** people who have experienced emotional abuse, perfectionism or legalistic religion. Fire and brimstone sermons can crush the heart and Jesus is asked into the heart out of fear. Perfectionists received love and praise

hen they did things right but harshly criticized for coming up short. Love then = being right all the time, which isn't going to happen! Body system = respiratory system. Can't breathe deeply or catch their breath.

10. **Trust Vs Control:** A study of common traits in Jesus, Lincoln, Gandhi, Mother Teresa found TRUST as the thread. Most trusted God more than people which helped their decision of people to trust. Body system is the reproductive so tied to sex struggles.

11. **Humility Vs Image Control:** Stems from a belief that if I'm not okay and if people get to know me, they will see that, so I need them to see a manufactured me instead of the real me. They take many steps and so much energy into this. Body system is circulatory

12. **Self-Control Vs Out of Control:** No self-control = can't love, realize our dreams, and often destroy our health. When self-control is done right it is effortless. Body system is the musculoskeletal system.

NEXT STEPS
Take the Heart Issues Finder.
Start with lower score and work on it until the emotion is below one. Work on the next lowest score.

After You Lower Scores on The Heart issues finder - go to the 12 categories
one per day and continue this maintenance for the rest of your life.

COMMON QUESTIONS:
What Should I expect to happen? A changed picture or memory you are focusing on in terms of emotions, but not the actual picture. Feeling of peace and closure.

What if I feel no progress?
If no Change after 5 attempts, look for another picture. Try the greatest intensity instead of the earliest time. If still no change, another issue may be tied to the root cause.

What if I feel worse after?
Like a physical detox, a mental detox can be uncomfortable for some as emotions are being cleared and issues are healed. It will stop when detox is complete.

How will I know if this is working?
You may feel a deeper sense of peace and that that things you often struggle with are less of a concern.

Sometimes I feel a battle going on inside myself. Why is that?
This is 'Conscious Conflict'. When you are not ready to let because it gives you comfort. i.e.: food, drugs, alcohol.

What if healing doesn't happen?
The first Place to look is your Heart. Be honest and ask if you have a conscious conflict? The second place to look is how you prayed. Do you choose a quiet, peaceful time and place? How often did you do the Daily CRUSH on the next page?

WEEK 9
Change Your Brain, Change Your Life

Your Automatic Thoughts

Your thoughts will determine whether you do or do not succeed with the goals you have set. Your thoughts must serve your plans for your life and your plans to help others. Your thoughts can be in YOUR control. There is saying we love, "Don't believe everything you think." Just because is passes through your mind does not make it true. Your thoughts must SERVE YOU and LIFT YOU UP, not harm you and keep you down. You can re-wire your brain to create winning thoughts that will help you build the life you desire and help others do the same. Do not skip through this section lightly, this is vital to your growth as a human while on this earth. This is vital to your ability to help others restore their health and lead them to a new lifestyle!

Be Careful of Your Thoughts!

When you think, chemicals are released. Those chemicals dictate how you 'feel'. Your brain receives information from the world within you just like it does from the world around you. We want you to have no limits in the exercise above so that you 'feel' a sensation of freedom. Feelings and emotions are converted into chemicals released into your blood. They inform you of trouble in your world or cause for celebration. They change the chemistry of every cell in your body, delivering the electric nerve impulses of whatever your brain is thinking and feeling. Your thoughts affect your energy moment to moment.

Emotion	Body Produces
Bliss and Love	Endorphins
Peace and tranquility	Valium
Acute Stress	Adrenaline
Chronic Stress	Cortisol
Exhilarated	Interleukin and Interferon

"The only reason a medication can have an effect on you is because your body already makes it naturally. That's why your brain cells have the receptor site for drugs to bind to. If your body did not make it, the cell receptor would not exist." — Bruce Lipton PhD

You have 45,000 - 51,000 thoughts a day.
For most individuals 80% of their thoughts are damaging and to make matters worse, 90% of them get carried forward to the next day's 51,000 thoughts.

- So, if you're thinking damaging thoughts, you'll cause yourself to think more damaging thoughts. This is not going to get you out of your mess. We have been taught to think that many of these 51,000 thoughts are "sub-conscious" thoughts. Affirmations make your sub-conscious thoughts conscious.

- If you begin making conscious empowering thoughts, you become more aware of the damaging thoughts that are threatening to take over. When you're not aware of your thoughts, they tend to be damaging and can induce a spiral downward.

Do you believe anything is attainable in your life?
- What blocks, if any come up when you do this exercise?
- What beliefs or messages are getting in the way of manifesting your dreams?

The Human Hard Drive
In the human computer, everything that ever happened to you was recorded in the form of memories. - your birth, your first bath, learning to walk, etc. Only 10% of the memories are conscious. 90% are subconscious or memories of the heart. All data is stored in our memories as images and that is how they are recalled. So, if you have wondered for years:

- why do I get angry when I shouldn't?
- Why do I eat when I'm trying to lose weight?
- Why do I think things I don't want to be thinking?
- Why am I sad for no reason?
- Why do I self-sabotage all the time?

"our internal images and how we order those images are our thoughts Human reasoning is always imagistic."
- Dr. Antonio DiMaggio MD PhD head of neurology at USC.

Whatever problems you have inside of you can exist as images and your associations are the neurology created by those energy patterns. The only way to heal them is with another energy pattern. The reason you have a short fuse is that you reactivate have unconscious memories and the feelings that are stored on your hard drive. The biggest problem with healing is convincing people to make the effort. The human body is a miracle in its resilience. I have seen people 100% recover from illness when I was not sure if they were going to be around next week. Why would the creator make emotional healing in the brain any different?

Plant and Nurture the Seeds to Success
Think about what you desire. How does that make you feel? If you feel good, describe your feelings below. If you don't feel good, ask, "Why does that cause me to feel bad?" When you are feeling bad, change your biology. You might throw your shoulders back, put a smile on your face, hum, sing, or even dance.

As you surround yourself with positive energy, you will find that circumstances, events, opportunities, and people will begin to appear in your life.

"Future medicine will be based on controlling energy in the body. "
- William killer Nobel prize laureate

What Will Fear of Success Cost You?

When I ask this, people look at me like "are you crazy, I don't fear success!" But there are people who have this fear and don't even realize it! They're in their 'comfort zone' and the thought of change is painful. They are unhealthy, unhappy, unfulfilled, lonely or broke but, change is hard. It takes work and they convince themselves or rationalize it and stay right where they are. So, be honest and ask yourself this question because this is real! **What Will Fear of Success Cost You?**

Now, the other side of the coin -- **What Will Fear of Failure Cost You?**

There Is More Energy in Love Than in Fear.

It's the highest-octane fuel available. (Not love for a person—love for *everyone*; for Life; for the Earth and everything in it. Live life in an ocean of love.) Most of us, live in an ocean of fear. Love is tireless, healing, inexhaustible and brings people together. It is powerful beyond measure and surpasses all understanding. Have you ever looked at the things you do and say and asked yourself, "Am I doing this from love, or am I doing this from fear?" This question is the most important choice you can make. It is the choice you were born to make each moment. Choosing to act with love no matter what is happening inside you (pain of fear) and around you (a national or international crisis) is creating authentic power. Choosing to fear almost always happens unconsciously. Choosing to love always happens consciously.

As you are learning in your Recreate Program - you have the ability to create the life you desire, but it begins with your thoughts. When you become aware of the state of your thought-life, you can see where you need to RECREATE your thoughts and redesign your life. We all have thoughts and behaviors we don't want and need to improve, so let's create a list. If you can't think of any then THINK HARDER! It's awesome to be happy with your life and I wish that for everyone. But no one reading this journal has reached their full potential. If you are happy and content with your life then ask yourself, "how can I help others to be the same? Who can I mentor in my life?" There's always room to become more and contribute more.

Doing It Right

We seldom focus on things that we like about ourselves, instead we linger over things we want to change. I want you to consider your positive attributes. Make an inventory of your best qualities, abilities and attributes. Are you a compassionate person? Put it down. Are you a hard worker? Write every quality down in a short sentence, beginning with "I AM, and I HAVE" and use the present tense. Examples:

- I AM a bright light in the world
- I HAVE grit and empathy
- I AM relentless
- I AM good with people
- I AM an example of what is possible.

These statements affirm who you are. An inventory will help you appreciate who you are and who you wish to become. These short prayers are highly useful to change our focus and conquer the Lies (self - doubt or fear) we hear or tell ourselves and help you succeed.

Write seven "I AM's" or "I HAVE's". These, along with your new beliefs above will become your prayers/meditations:

1.

_____

2.

_____

3.

_____

4.

_____

5.

_____

6.

_____

7.

_____

Match your attributes to your goals.
Which of the favorable qualities that you listed above will help you accomplish your goals? If want to stop overeating, then draw on your strong will to be stubborn. You might need to draw on the fact that you are caring and need to be the example for your loved ones. Or that you are intelligent.

Make your prayers/meditations visible so you use them. Repetition is the key to making them effective so practice thinking them many times a day:

1. Write your prayers in a journal every morning when you get up and every night before bed.

2. Meditate on them. Ideally, first thing you think of when you get up and the last before you turn in.

3. Shut your eyes, block out the rest of the world. Say and repeat the words but consider what the words mean to you; consider the future and try to feel the emotion that the prayers bring up.

4. Leave reminders in assorted places on sticky notes and leave them where you'll see them: - where you sit at the kitchen table, tape to your car steering wheel, slip one on or PC monitor, etc. Every time you see the note, read it and consider it.

5. Carry them with you. Put it in your phone notes. If you need a pick-me-up, or find you are wavering, read them.

Mind Controls Matter Science has proven that we are programmed for love and have a natural bias for optimism. The Creator gave us the power of love to overcome fear. According to Eric R. Kandel, your thoughts reach your DNA and can turn your genes on and off, transforming the structure of brain cells (neurons). Thinking will change your brain structure. Your focus dictates the release of chemicals which in turn build proteins which alter our brain's wiring and function.

This is fantastic news for those with bad genetics! To switch on your brain, you have to address the lies of- society, the masses, the media – these influences who say 'it's impossible' or 'it's not worth it' or 'you are not worthy' etc. The creator wants you to conquer your Giant Lies that keep you from making an impact on the world and keep you from your purpose. Be YOU. - Fight your battle how the Divine designed you, with your gifts and blessings, not like someone else.

WEEK 10

Triggers for a NEW YOU!

Once you have completed your Daily CRUSH Exercise for 21 days straight, you have created a new pattern in your brain. In this week you will learn the power of 'triggers' to replace old thoughts and actions with new ones. Let's get started!

3 Steps to Recreate Your Brain so that your thoughts serve you:

1. **DECIDE TO CHANGE YOUR THOUGHTS**
    Eliminate thoughts that hurt you or limit you and replace them with new thoughts that work in your favor.

2. **AUTOMATIZE YOUR NEW THOUGHTS**
    to become a natural reflex. You have to perform mental repetitions just like exercising your muscles at the gym.

3. **ACT ON YOUR NEW THOUGHTS**
    You already decided to change your thoughts by taking that first step months ago
    to begin your own health journey when you began your Recreate Program. So now, we will help you design many new thoughts that serve your growth. For your new thoughts to become 'automatic' you must practice and develop the skills to overcome your old habits. Here you will find examples of exercises to begin re-wiring your brain so that your thoughts work IN your favor and you begin designing the thought-life that you desire! Then you will get a chance to write your own triggers!

Are you experiencing anything in your life that you do not feel you deserve? Most often this is something that does not seem "fair."

Reflect and ask what part you have played in attracting it to you. Be honest and be careful not to see yourself as a victim. Write down your thoughts:

Prayer and meditation are the best ways to change your thoughts but, it is required daily. Every day you are being bombarded by the media, society and people around us every day with energy and frequencies that do not serve you or your goals.

Prayer is like a daily mental detox to renew your mind. This is why we created the daily CRUSH exercise. The frequency you transmit goes out instantly with consistent power. **How does knowing this change your perspective about the power of your thoughts and feelings?**

Triggering New Behaviors Exercise

Create new daily routines in two steps:
1. Look for triggers or cues that already exist in your life's daily routine.
2. The KEY to a new behavior is to insert the new behavior after an existing one.

Morning Behaviors

Existing Behavior - Trigger		New Behavior
When I	Weigh myself	I will	Take my vitamins
When I	Brush my teeth	I will	Drink 24 ounces of water
When I	Have my coffee	I will	Do morning magic and Daily CRUSH

Now it's your turn. Fill in the template with existing behaviors and new behaviors:

New Morning Behaviors

Existing Behavior - Trigger		New Empowering Behavior
When I	I will	
When I	I will	
When I	I will	

Evening Examples Behaviors

Existing Behavior – Trigger		New Empowering Behavior
When I	Come home	I will	Kiss and hug my family
When I	Change my work clothes	I will	Spend quality time with my wife, my kids, etc....
When I	Go to bed	I will	Journal things I failed so I can succeed tomorrow

Evening Behaviors

Existing Behavior – Trigger		New Empowering Behavior
When I	I will	
When I	I will	
When I	I will	

Behavior Triggers Become Rituals

Now that you have new triggers for new, empowering behaviors you can take them to the next level and create an entire ritual.

EXAMPLE RITUAL	Get out of bed and make coffee	Brush teeth and Pray →	20 - ozs. of water →	Take morning vitamin pack →	Drink coffee → Read inspirational or bible message
CREATE YOUR OWN RITUAL					

Weekly Wellness Warrior:

Let's build your discipline muscles that you have already started with the Morning Magic, Daily Crush, Evening Magic by adding Weekly Warriors! To live a life that is exceptional you must be exceptional and do the things that others rarely do.

Complete RARE every week:

- **R**andom Acts of Kindness
- **A**nticipate: Future out and plan what is ahead for you to win.
- **R**esults: Never be surprised by what happens.
- **E**xpectation: Create the destiny that allows you to win.

Random Act of Kindness: Do something kind for someone:

- Can't be an act you already currently do.
- Something outside of your normal routine.
  i.e., buy a coffee for someone in line behind you, do a chore you normally do not, help a senior with yardwork.

Anticipate Future out and plan ahead for you to WIN
- Birthday party on Wed, stay on clean eating
- Late night on Wed so set alarm a little later, but don't hit snooze
- Business meeting with boss, change my mindset to winning not complaining
- Thurs am workout is key to staying disciplined

Results I am not surprised by the outcomes
- Felt energized at birthday party, made new friends and came home feeling on fire!
- Woke up without hitting snooze, got dressed and out the door.
- Brought my new idea to my boss and she loved it! I am the lead on the project!!
- Killed my work out because I wrote in my journal that discipline is the key to freedom.

Expectation Create the plan that allows you to win
- Eat big salad before birthday party so I'm not hungry
- Compete my journal exercises so I wake up ready to win the day
- Before meeting with boss, do a power prayer to build my confidence
- Get up, even if I'm tired, drink coffee to help my workout at the gym'

Write your RARE here:

Random Act of Kindness

_____

_____

_____

_____

Anticipation

_____

_____

_____

_____

_____

Results

_____

_____

_____

_____

_____

Expectation

_____

_____

_____

_____

_____

The Success Cycle:

This is pretty self-explanatory but don't let the simplicity cause you to underestimate the importance of it. Everything starts with your potential which is the gifts you have been blessed with. In order for humanity to evolve as it should, we need to be using our gifts to their fullest. When we don't shine our bright light in the world, everyone loses out. Our family, our friends, co-workers our community and the repercussions are felt further then you know.

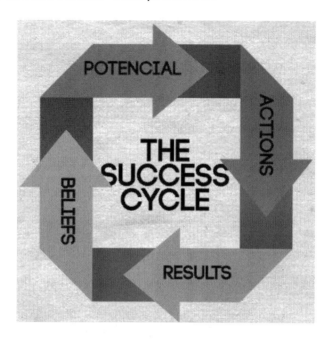

WEEK 11

The Power of Relationships

The biggest thing that keeps people from having a relationship they want is that they're looking for a relationship to be the solution to their problems. This approach tends to disempower both people in a relationship. Think of a relationship as a place to give rather than a place to get.

1. **5 Stages of Relationships:** credit Logan Stout
   i. **Honeymoon stage:** everything is perfect.
   ii. **Adversity**: some quit here, some progress and push ahead. Ever hear of Steve Jobs? Yes. Warren Buffet? Yes.   Brandon Zychowski? No. Why? Because he quit.
   iii. **Progress:** moving forward to deepen the bond of the relationship. Don't let arguments get out-of-control – use pattern interrupts on each other. Be playful!
   iv. **Management Mode:** this is where potential goes to die. Enthusiasm wanes, then negative associations are created which are the primary killers of relationships.
   A marriage on life support. Ask, what can I do for my queen to be her king? (or vice versa). How can I court her like when we dated?
   v. **Freedom:** ultimate trust. No concerns about who spouse is talking to, where they are, etc.

2. **Love Language**s
Gary Chapman wrote about the 5 languages that make us feel truly, loved. We are all a hybrid but, one resonates more than others. Finding the right language is the key to helping a person feel loved. This is not just for a spouse. It includes parents, child, girlfriend, friends, etc. Remember the 'good ole days' when 'experts' told us to treat all our children the same to prevent jealousy? Yet children still felt their

siblings were loved more. Love languages explains why. Using myself and my family as examples will comprehend each *love language* more clearly.

Here are the 5 Love Languages:

i. Words: To love them is to talk to them. Our oldest fell in this category as a child. Our words and our tone meant a lot. When we reprimanded her, we had to be careful with our tone whereas her sister needs a strong tone. But for her, we just had to tell her what she did wrong. We used to say she is "so sensitive," but now, we know that she hears what and how we say it more clearly. When I say, "I love you," she knows we mean it.

ii. Time: To love them is to spend time with them. For my youngest daughter, she needs attention. She always wants to play games, bounce on the trampoline or go for a bike ride. It's important for her to be with people that love her. It is not that she is needy, she just needs to connect every day.

iii. Gifts: When they look at the gift they think, "this person thinks of me and loves me." As my oldest matured her language changed to cherish gifts from those she loves, and it had nothing to do with monetary value. It could be a shell found on a beach. For her it's important to "see" the love.

iv. Acts of Service: to love them is to do things for them." For my wife, when I help tidy up and cook for her, this speaks volumes of love to her. It's not the same if she has to ask, it has to be a spontaneous thought on my part, thinking, "hey, I know she will like it if I do this for her!"

v. Touch: Without kisses and hugs, they feel unloved. When my wife and I started dating, we always snuggled as we talked or watched TV and we still touch and hold hands. I anticipate we will be one of those cute couples in our 90's when we will still 'smooch' in public. At least I hope so :)

3. Nothing of lasting and measurable value in life can be created without absolute commitment:

i. Identify and write down exactly what you want in a relationship

ii. Write down what you don't want in a relationship

iii.   Identify what the relationship needs to be for you to be happy with yourself and contribute to it in an effective way

4. Want your relationships to last? Do the following:

i.   Find out their love language and meet it consistently. Use this link to take the quiz.
https://www.5lovelanguages.com/quizzes/

ii.   Ask questions that encourage Love 🖤 to be expressed. Give what they most to receive and don't get trapped by "you do it first and then I will"

iii.   Be spontaneous to creating special moments with enthusiasm to enhance your relationship

iv.   develop a list of unique things you can do together to enhance your relationship on an ongoing basis.

WEEK 12

Thoughts = Energy!

We started this journal with energy so it's only fitting to end that way.

Energy from the view of your soul is very different than energy from your five senses. For the senses, energy is the ability to get things done. The more you have, the more things you accomplish. The questions are:

- How much energy do you have?
- How is your sleep?
- How is your stress?
- Did you follow your ideal diet and take your supplements?
- Are your cells healthy?

The problem is physical or mental. People go to doctors, nutritionists and counsellors for this kind of energy. From the perspective of your soul, the question is not 'how much', but 'what kind' of energy you have. There are two kinds of energy:

1. **FEAR:** Anger, jealousy, guilt, stress, cravings and addictions *feel* like different energies. Each has its own sensation (pain) and a specific consequence (destructive - painful). They feel different, but they are only different experiences of one energy: fear.

2. **LOVE.** Different experiences feel like different energies. i.e.: patience, peace, kindness, self-control. Each has its own sensation (feel good) and a specific consequence (health and joy). While they feel different, they are only different experiences of one energy: love.

It gets interesting when Fear appears as Love. For example, romantic love. You long for someone (pain), try to influence them (pain) attract them into your life (pleasure), but pain follows when they leave or die. Drama is created when fear appears as love. It's painful and destructive because it is not love. There are many examples of fear appearing as love. Care providers or clergy may appear loving and yet some act to feel better about themselves. When their efforts are not appreciated or even rejected, they are disappointed (pain), unappreciated (pain) and resentment (pain) grows and becomes anger (pain). When the bottom-line reason for an action is for another, the energy is love. When the bottom-line, reason is for yourself, the energy is fear. Only you can know your real intention, and you may not know it unless you have the courage to look for it and find it.

The Law of Attraction – Like Attracts Like. It's a universal law. Change your frequency and you change your life. The Secret was the first movie to popularize the Law of Attraction. If you have not seen it, watch it on Netflix. Why is it that we duplicate patterns and draw the same sort of friends or lovers?

"The human brain emits frequencies, which when focused, are picked up by other human brains, and affect other physical matter."
- Caroline Leaf PhD

Our vibration is neutral – BUT if you believe all men are cheaters -- all jobs lead nowhere --- you will always be poor ... you attract those experiences into our life. The media, society, television .... is forever flooding us with images of fear, anger and bad news that is most often, completely out of proportion to reality, because let's face it, their job is to stir your emotions. That causes a lot of unnecessary worry and doomsayers. Be aware of the energy you put out, as it is like a calling signal or lighthouse drawing the same vibration back to you. If you get jealous or mad, if you're petty or judgmental, it's likely that you'll call in others who mimic this energy toward you.

YOUR BRAIN IS A TRANSMITTER
Your brain is the most powerful transmitter and receiver of information. Just the mind activity from you reading these next few lines generates electromagnetic, electrochemical and quantum action in your brain cells (neurons).

- Magnetic fields that can be measured.
- Electrical impulses that can be tracked.
- You emit Photons that can be captured on computer screens.
- Vibrations in the membranes of your neurons can be measured.

These signals can come from inside your body (emotional, biochemical and spiritual). Or from the outside your body - food toxins, social network, and nurturing you receive. - Pennisi. "Behind the Science of Gene Expression", Science (2001).

In a family that suffers from Cancer, the propensity of Cancer is the same in ADOPTED KIDS AS it is in the biological children.   -- Bruce Lipton, PHD

Are we just failing to understand physics – or is there more to it?
Einstein and Tesla recognized that people do not understand their equations or its ramifications. Since 1999 Serge Benhayon has been teaching the concepts as stated by Einstein and Tesla. They combined science, religion and philosophy of $E=mc^2$ and how it applies to life. The implications that everything is energy means:

- Everything is connected – nothing is separate in the entire universe.
- Everything happens because energy makes it so - no random chance or accident.

- We are energetic beings in communion with the universe and we have a sixth sense that feels everything.
- Every choice has a consequence – we are affected by the way we live.
- Death can't be the end. Energy can't be destroyed – we change from form to formlessness.
- True freedom = awareness of the energy we choose - it gives us the quality of our thoughts, actions and choices.

WHY? In the past 100 years, why has society chosen to …
1. Ignore, deny, resist and reject these understandings.

2. Fail to apply them in our daily lives

3. Go as far as to ridicule and even attack those who expand upon them?

- How long before we realize who we are, what we are a part of?

- Could it be that these understandings bring a responsibility that most are not ready or willing to accept?

- What if we could no longer blame others – realizing that we are connected to everything that happens to us?

Everything Vibrates at Different Frequencies.
Every cell, every organ in your body … everything is energy. Everything is made of the same atoms. The only thing that differentiates them is the frequencies at which they vibrate. This determines their material make up. Your thinking creates a powerful signal that passes to your cells and enters your DNA that is dormant and zipped up like a cocoon until activated by the signal. When activated it opens the cocoon and

the DNA code is read by RNA that photocopies the code to build proteins. This is called 'Genetic Expression'.

- Kandell, E. et al. "Molecular biology of Memory". Essentials of Neuroscience and Behavior 1995

What thoughts do you send out to the world? When you vibrate at a certain level, the whole universe conspires and creates events that work to create your life. The Law of Attraction says that whatever vibration you put out, attracts similar vibrations. **What transmissions have you put out into the universe that worked for you? Make a list.**

YOUR brain has the power to create and transmit any frequency you want. The frequency of your transmission is key. You must powerfully and consistently transmit out to the world.
Write down something (or things) that you want to manifest in your life.

How do they support your goals?

How Often Are You Transmitting per day?

1   2   3   4   5   6   7   8   9   10

Remember, whatever frequency you emit — that same frequency is drawn to you magnetically. This is a law of the universe. **Write down the transmissions that you wish to emit into the people around you?**

How do they support your goals?

Worry = Negative Goal Setting.
It is the opposite of faith. When you worry you are literally - **Praying in Reverse!**

By thinking and dwelling on what you hope will not happen you give it your energy and you make it bigger. You are actually channeling your faith into what you don't want to happen. Make a list of things you constantly worry about and follow them with a new statement of hope and faith.

Example:
If you are in debt your worry is, "Right now I'm in debt and it is stressful."

followed with,

"I have no idea how I'm going to get out of debt, but I know something will present itself. I don't know how, but I have faith that I will be overcome this."

In the blank pages at the back of this journal, list the Things You Worry About and the Hope and Faith Statements.

People have thoughts they want something, but that "something" is beyond their reach until the tipping point occurs. When the positive ball becomes larger than the negative ball.

Rate how large your ball of negativity was when you started this program:

1   2   3   4   5   6   7   8   9   10

Rate where your negative ball of energy is now:

1   2   3   4   5   6   7   8   9   10

WEEK 13

Action = Energy!

"Between every event in our lives and our response to that event is a space. In that space we make a choice. The choices we make defines our character. Viktor Frankl, MD

How You Respond to 'Negative' Events in Your Life

Ok, so now you can see you have a choice. All events are neutral. They are not positive or negative. YOU assign the meaning to them. The short time between the event and the interpretation we make in our brain has all the power to make you or break you. It will determine the path you set for entire direction that your life will take. If you have children, they are watching your choices, what will you model for them? Are you going to model giving up when things get difficult, or are you going to model that yes life is not fair, but you get up and do the best you can. So, think about your choices every day, keep telling yourself your family is watching, you kids, your spouse, your friends. What choices do you want them to make when their lives become difficult? Say it out loud. - do you want them to give up or do you want them to go on despite adversity?

Changing Your Story

We like to think we can live however and get away with being reckless, irresponsible and harsh. That we can eat whatever we want, drink alcohol, take drugs, watch porn, argue and/or fight, be corrupt, greedy - and not be accountable. BUT, for every energetic action, there is an equal reaction. Change the narrative of your challenges and think about what is the meaning of your challenge? What is the gift?

Reclaim Your Faith

Empowerment is associated with a reconciled identity and coherence. "Holding on" to previous social roles and identities can take control of you, and the process of letting go of your identity as a sick, tired, fat, depressed person into a whole and healthy person means "Letting go", and thereby learning to identify and accept the new boundaries and possibilities.

You need to decide in advance so you can reverse engineer this process to work in your favor. Decide right now that everything evolves perfectly. You may not understand why a "negative" event is perfect but, Faith says you don't need to. Faith says it is all designed perfectly to move you in the direction you want your life to take even if it does not appear that way in the moment.

ASSIGNMENT:

STEP 1. Pay attention to everything you say today.
Are your words negative or positive? Choose words wisely. Use them to instantly change your thoughts. When someone asks you how you feel, say something to make you feel better.

i.e., "I feel terrible, but I'm working through it and just telling you that, I'm already feeling better."

Here are some phrases to practice using every chance you get:

- Everything always works out for me
- I AM blessed.
- This appears to be negative, but it will all work out fine.
- Everything works out to my advantage in the end.
- I expect miracles, and I get miracles.

STEP 2. I Am Responsible for The Condition of my Life.
When fully understood – these awakenings are the key to empowerment and freedom. You are no longer a victim and you come to a deeper understanding to realize you have the power to transform and truly heal and live a life way beyond anything you ever imagined

was possible. You can put an end to the suffering you feel has been inflicted on you and the thing is, you don't have to take our word for it! The great thing about the energetic truth is that when you walk it out in your life it makes a massive difference – you feel it in your body, so you know the truth of it for yourself. Your experience in your mind, body and spirit reveals and confirms the energetic truth. Do not deny and ignore these understandings, for you will only perpetuate separation and suffering. Incorporating them into your life and into the world gives you the power to transform EVERYTHING. You will affect a deep amount of healing within yourself, your community if we truly align and apply the energetic truth.

STEP 3. Recall 4 of Your Greatest Successes:
In the pages at the back of the journal, write a paragraph describing each one. Use these examples to remind yourself that you can always find a way.

STEP 4. Lighten up!
One positive thought is more potent than 10,000 negative ones so your positive energy can transform an entire group of negative people.

The moment you change your vibration, everything starts reversing.
Physical changes may take time to manifest, but energy changes immediately. Next time you find yourself in a so-called negative experience or feel like a victim of someone's anger, stop and take a breath to look at the role you played. Release the emotions and choose empowering thoughts instead. Search for gifts from the experience. How did this serve you? How did it make you feel?

This may be difficult, but it will shift the energy in a positive way. You will know you mastered this when something goes wrong in your life, and can honestly say, "I don't know why, but this is going to work to my advantage." Do you see your role in that creation? You are the creator of your life.

When you MASTER these principles, you can predict and create your future. Choosing to accept full responsibility for your life means you never blame others for what happens to you. It also means you have full control of your destiny. In reading those words, write down any thoughts or feelings that arise in you:

TWO CHOICES: Holding on and Letting go.
1. **Holding on**: think about your social roles and identities you hold. They are the essence of who you are. A parent, a sibling, a realtor, a role model. Who do you hang out with? your peer group, social group, extended family, your church – who can facilitate coping, and staying motivated in your health?

So, the quality of your community really matters. Because the reality is, we do what our friends do. If they do disease promoting stuff, that is what we do. If we get friends who do health promoting stuff, that is what we will do.

2. **Letting go**: Ask yourself, do your friends support health promoting behaviors or disease promoting behaviors? What do they create in your life?

Match Your Actions with your thoughts

When you match your actions and your thoughts the universe will deliver you amazing circumstances toward the outcomes you are desiring in your life. However, if you proceed with action before you have aligned your thoughts, there is not enough action in the world to make any real difference. Develop the skill of alignment and you will discover the power of Inspired Action.

From experience, we want you to know that connection to something higher than yourself is critical to the success of your thought - life. Whatever your belief is, whatever you may call that over-riding force of the universe- God, Spirit, Source, Mother Nature, etc.- all this work will fall flat if you do not truly connect through these exercises with that power. If you are struggling in this area and feel you have no direction, reach out for help- we are here for you.

We have learned helplessness vs owning that we have control. That we can hold on to the essential parts of ourselves, and that we can find meaning in our circumstances, however they are. The power of creating self-talk, remembering that what you say out loud and in your head your body will make come true. Prayers are incredibly powerful. A social network can either promote the adoption of disease

promoting behavior or health promoting behavior. Having a mission statement, so you understand what your higher purpose is, can dramatically improve your resilience.

The GRIT FACTOR

The Grit Factor is essential to reaching your goals in all aspects of your life. Do you have it? We want you to know that if you have it or not, it can be attained by anyone. We are products of a growing Grit Factor. Prior to knowing exactly what our goals were with Wellness Method, we were just coasting along comfortably - but when we saw a way to reach more people and really change lives, we went after it and had to build a lot of Grit along the way.

Logan Stout, a dear friend and mentor of the Wellness Method is the author of "The Grit Factor" (and CEO of ID Life). Logan explains what the Grit Factor is …

"It is your ability to see what you want, understand what you don't want, and let nothing get in the way of your goals. You will experience hardships and challenges along the way to any goal. If you have a high Grit Factor you will persevere and hit your target."

To have a high Grit Factor, you must possess some foundations:

1. You understand your mind is a 'goal achieving machine'.

2. Your goals or targets must excite you!

3. You must believe you can achieve your goals.

4. Your goals will grow bigger and bolder as you grow.

5. Your goals need your daily attention.

6. You need a goal for every aspect of your life.

7. You're never stagnant.

8. Your habits move you toward your goals, not away from them.

WEEK 14

LIFECYCLES

One Life Cycle = 365 Days
In one year, you will replace 98% of the cells in your body. However, if you add at least one, 30 - day Brain Surgery, you can actually replace close to 100% OF THE CELLS IN YOUR BODY!

What Will Your New Model Look Like Compared to One Year Ago?
Look back, look at how far you have come and celebrate your growth! People make new year's resolutions every year that on average die within 2 weeks. I don't want to diminish them in any way, after all, at least they are trying. In 365 days, you can crush every New Year's resolution you have made for the past 10, 15 or even 20 years for some people. You have the road map to accomplish all of your goals in one year of RECREATE! potential How good will it feel to knock them out of the park and bring yourself to a whole new potential waiting for you on the other side?

SEASONS OF CHANGE -- 4 Seasons in one year.

A season of change = one 30-day brain surgery. After you completed your 30 days, choose at least one to at the most three thoughts to change. For most people, they have more than that to cover so, we suggest a 10 break after completing one season before starting the next one. This will allow some time to rest your brain and let it download and really sink into a deeper level of your subconscious. After 10 days you can start on your next brain surgery and when you break down the numbers you will find that you can perform 5 brain surgeries per year. That is an awesome amount of change!

So, not only do you transform your physical health, but you can also completely your transformation by adding the brain surgeries to fully RECREATE yourself in one year. Here is how it breaks down:

- One season = 90 Days.
    - 30 brain surgery
    - 30 days of Morning Magic + Daily Crush + Evening Magic
    - 30 Days of Weekly Warriors

This Allows you 4 Brain Surgeries Every Year.
YOU choose how many brain surgeries you want to do each year. Your decision will come down to how many changes you want to make and how much growth you want in your life.

Lifecycles: Your Accountability Structure for all aspects of your life.

Level 1: 30 Day Brain surgery.

Level 2: Morning Magic - Daily Crush – Evening Magic

Level 3: RARE - Weekly Wellness Warrior

Level 4: 1 Mastery LIFECYLE - 4 Seasons

OUR PERSONAL CHALLENGE TO YOU

1. **For the next 10 days,**
   Review the past 13 weeks and do any assignments or other work that you have not yet completed.

2. **Master your mindset.**
   Continue to do your daily CRUSH and RAER Weekly Warriors for the next 4 weeks.

3. **Create Your Life!**

   What would make you SPARKLE? If you were guaranteed success, what would your life look like? Use the SPARKLE template at the back of your journal to help track your growth in different areas of your life. Have inspiring goals to drive you to SPARKLe.

The Pursuit of Happiness

In the Pursuit of Happiness, Martin Seligman studied happiness using Confucius, Aristotle, and modern psychology theories and found that the most satisfied of people were those who had discovered and exploited their unique combination of signature strengths such as humanity, temperance, and persistence. He also found that happiness has 3 dimensions that can be intentionally created.

3 Levels

Level 1: The Pleasant Life:

The first level is where we appreciate basic pleasures as:
- Companionship of friends and family, lovers and spouses.
- the natural environment.
- our physical, bodily needs.

Level 2: The Good Life:

The next level is achieved through discovering your unique virtues and strengths and employing them creatively to enhance your own personal life.

Level 3: The Meaningful Life:

The highest level is achieved by employing your unique strengths for a purpose greater than ourselves.

Reassess your goals

At least once a year reflect on the year ahead and what areas of your life that you want to experience personal growth that will make your life SPARKLe!

Find your tribe.

Surround yourself with positive people that have faith in you and that support your goals. You are the result of the people that you have in your life. So, in 5, 10 20 years from now ask yourself, how will those people influence your life?

How to Solve Problems Quickly

Use this system to solve problems effectively: credit to Tony Robbins

1. **Manage your emotions:**
   Disappointment, frustration, doubt, etc.... Acknowledge your feelings and the message they are sending but too many people get stuck here. It's okay to feel bad sometimes, everyone does but you need something to anchor yourself. If you don't have an anchor you will get tossed by the storms that will happen in your life. Faith is your anchor. Faith in the Creator and faith in yourself.

   Too many people ask how are you feeling? Feelings change by the minute. A better question is how is your faith?

2. **Write the problem down.**
   Spend 10% of your time on the problem and 90% on the solution. Create a plan to handle the problem using the following questions:

i. What is great about this problem?
Every problem is an opportunity to learn something new!

ii. What's not perfect yet?

iii. What am I willing to do to make it the way I want it?

iv. What am I willing to no longer do to make it the way I want it?

v. How can I enjoy the process?

3. **Observe if it is working.**
If it is working great, if not change your approach.

4. **If it still is not working, get help!**
Find an expert, a mentor or coach to help you find solutions.

SPIRITUAL TEMPLATE

Align your Core Purpose with the Universe	Exercises: Power Meditation Journaling Daily CRUSH Triggers		
Spiritual Exercise		**Time**	**Breakthroughs**
Example Day	Power Meditation	20 minutes	I felt God speak to me in my heart
Day 1			
Day 2			
Day 3			
Day 4			
Day 5			
Day 6			
Day 7			

DIET TEMPLATE

Diet	Portion sizes in ounces? Baked, Boiled, Grilled, Fried or Zapped? Brand Name?				
	Breakfast	**Snack**	**Lunch**	**Snack**	**Dinner**
Example Day	Smoothie	Apple	Lean Protein Healthy Fat Fibrous Carb	Carrots and avocado	Lean Protein Healthy fat Fibrous Carb
Day 1					
Day 2					
Day 3					
Day 4					
Day 5					
Day 6					
Day 7					

EXERCISE

	Metabolic Bursts	Resistance Exercise	Stretching
Example Day	Jumping Jacks, Burpees, Lunges	Free weights, Nautilus Machines, Tubing.	Neck, legs, back, hips, shoulders,
Day 1			
Day 2			
Day 3			
Day 4			
Day 5			
Day 6			
Day 7			

SLEEP

Time asleep		# of times awakened Mins / Hours awake	Time awake Time got up		Naps per day
Example Day	9:30 10 pm	1: 5 mins	5am	5:15 am	10 mins
Day 1					
Day 2					
Day 3					
Day 4					
Day 5					
Day 6					
Day 7					

ATTITUDE = ALTITUDE

The lenses you look through to assign meaning the world and situations that arise in your life.		**Exercises:** Meditation Daily CRUSH	Journal Triggers
	Life Situation	**Old Attitude**	**New Attitude**
Example Day	Co-worker brings a box of donuts to work (or you see a commercial for donuts).	Those look amazing! I ate 2 and now I feel regret. I'm tired and my stomach hurts.	I remembered my WHY and I reflect on it. I also reflect on how great I feel when eating clean.
Example Day	My spouse criticized me.	My feelings are hurt, they always do this to me, it's not fair! I never criticize my spouse.	No one can control how I feel. Only I control that. Maybe they are going through something and need more support.

Day 1			
Day 2			
Day 3			
Day 4			
Day 5			
Day 6			
Day 7			

RELATIONSHIPS

	What am I creating in the lives around me?		
	Spouse/Partner	**Family -** parents, siblings, kids, etc..	**Community** (work, church, friends)
Example Day	I complimented my partner today and she smiled. I can see how she needs affirmations and it felt good!	I created stress in my kid's life because I was tired and had a short fuse. When my day is chaotic, I see that I take it out on my kids.	When I do my daily CRUSH and write in my journal, I feel so great when I get to work. I have more to give to my team!
Day 1			
Day 2			
Day 3			
Day 4			
Day 5			
Day 6			
Day 7			

KNOWLEDGE

	Internship	Certifications	Degrees
What do I need to learn to achieve what I want to in my life?			
Example Day	I want a real world experience from a mentor I trust and respect.	I need to have something that says I am an expert in a certain area"	I need a degree that allows me to legally perform the things I want to do.
Day 1			
Day 2			
Day 3			
Day 4			
Day 5			
Day 6			
Day 7			

LIVELIHOOD (Financial Wellness)

	Income	Expenses	My Portfolio
What is my relationship like with money?			
Examp le Day	I have a fixed income and I find myself saying far too often, "I can't afford that."	I am good at tracking my expenses. I live by, "It's not about how much money you make, it's about how much you keep!"	I find myself working a lot to build someone else's empire and yet I am not building my own. I want to change.
Day 1			
Day 2			
Day 3			
Day 4			
Day 5			
Day 6			
Day 7			

Educator

	Contribution	Generational Curses	Wealth
What am I creating in my life to leave a legacy for my family, my friends and my community?			
Example Day	I created a dream board & dream journal with my children, and we went through the SPARKLE steps.	I busted a Diabetes myth. I taught my children their choices determine their health not their genetics.	I created a wealth education plan to teach my community about financial wellness.
Day 1			
Day 2			
Day 3			
Day 4			
Day 5			
Day 6			
Day 7			

DAILY CRUSH
Reminder and Templates

Capture: Read a paragraph, verse or small section	Read a paragraph, verse or section of the book of your choice and <u>capture</u> a small portion of what you read that seems to be getting your attention. Something positive, uplifting, inspiring or healthy. When we "capture," the amygdala in our brain provides input to the mind about the emotions connected to the thoughts.
Reflect: Focus on the small section and write it down.	Find 3 - 5 words or a short phrase from the passage that you read above that really stand out for you. When we "reflect" the thalamus and hypothalamus provide motivation.
Unite: Write down those 3 - 5 words in the section to activate the brain. Write them 3 times	Write out those 3-5 words/phrase three times. Be sure these words are inspiring or uplifting in some way. When we "write," the central hub in our brains integrates everything to consolidate our thoughts. MRI's showed increased neural activity in large sections of the brain to sharpen the gray matter sharp, so we think "more positively" to activate thinking, healing and memory.
Silence: Take 5 minutes to go inside and then write you observations about what you learned.	Ask yourself and the Creator/Universe/Source, "What do you want me to hear?" Be silent and meditate on the phrase while being open to hearing The heart is a checking station to help us hear a new healthy thought to replace old toxic ones. Record in your journal or templates what you have 'heard' from your reflection on the phrase you wrote down. Use the blank pages in the back of your journal for this exercise
Healthy Acts: How did I use and implement the passage I reflected upon today?	Put it into action in your daily life. Whatever you learned and observed from the passage you reflected upon, implement it into your daily life. This is where we practice using new healthy thoughts until it becomes automatic. This is where your words and actions line up with your new thoughts, beliefs and feelings. This happens in the limbic system and makes you feel that the new thought is true. This is where your mind-heart congruence occurs. By using the new thought at least 7 times a day for 21 days, we can ingrain it into our brains and replace the old toxic thought forever.

RARE WEEKLY WARRIORS

Random Act of Kindness:	• One nice gesture you can do for someone that is not something you normally would do
Anticipation:	• Anticipation: Future out what is ahead for the win.
Expectation:	• Expectation: Create a plan that allows you to win.
Results:	• Results: Never be surprised by what happens.

WEEK 1: WEEKLY WARRIORS

Random Act of Kindness:	
Anticipation:	
Results:	
Expectation:	

Daily Crush: Day 1

Template

Capture: Read a paragraph, verse or small section	
Reflect: Focus on the small section and write it down.	
Unite: Write down those 3 - 5 words in the section to activate the brain. Write them 3 times	
Silence: Take 5 minutes to go inside and then write you observations about what you learned.	
Healthy Acts: How did I use and implement the passage I reflected upon today?	

Daily Crush: Day 2

Capture: Read a paragraph, verse or small section	
Reflect: Focus on the small section and write it down.	
Unite: Write down those 3 - 5 words in the section to activate the brain. Write them 3 times	
Silence: Take 5 minutes to go inside and then write you observations about what you learned.	
Healthy Acts: How did I use and implement the passage I reflected upon today?	

Daily Crush: Day 3

Capture: Read a paragraph, verse or small section	
Reflect: Focus on the small section and write it down.	
Unite: Write down those 3 - 5 words in the section to activate the brain. Write them 3 times	
Silence: Take 5 minutes to go inside and then write you observations about what you learned.	
Healthy Acts: How did I use and implement the passage I reflected upon today?	

Daily Crush: Day 4

Capture: Read a paragraph, verse or small section	
Reflect: Focus on the small section and write it down.	
Unite: Write down those 3 - 5 words in the section to activate the brain. Write them 3 times	
Silence: Take 5 minutes to go inside and then write you observations about what you learned.	
Healthy Acts: How did I use and implement the passage I reflected upon today?	

Daily Crush: Day 5

Capture: Read a paragraph, verse or small section	
Reflect: Focus on the small section and write it down.	
Unite: Write down those 3 - 5 words in the section to activate the brain. Write them 3 times	
Silence: Take 5 minutes to go inside and then write you observations about what you learned.	
Healthy Acts: How did I use and implement the passage I reflected upon today?	

Daily Crush: Day 6

Capture: Read a paragraph, verse or small section	
Reflect: Focus on the small section and write it down.	
Unite: Write down those 3 - 5 words in the section to activate the brain. Write them 3 times	
Silence: Take 5 minutes to go inside and then write you observations about what you learned.	
Healthy Acts: How did I use and implement the passage I reflected upon today?	

Daily Crush: Day 7

Capture: Read a paragraph, verse or small section	
Reflect: Focus on the small section and write it down.	
Unite: Write down those 3 - 5 words in the section to activate the brain. Write them 3 times	
Silence: Take 5 minutes to go inside and then write you observations about what you learned.	
Healthy Acts: How did I use and implement the passage I reflected upon today?	

WEEK 2 WEEKLY WARRIORS

Random Act of Kindness:	
Anticipation:	
Expectation:	
Results:	

Daily Crush: Day 8

Capture: Read a paragraph, verse or small section	
Reflect: Focus on the small section and write it down.	
Unite: Write down those 3 - 5 words in the section to activate the brain. Write them 3 times	
Silence: Take 5 minutes to go inside and then write you observations about what you learned.	
Healthy Acts: How did I use and implement the passage I reflected upon today?	

Daily Crush: Day 9

Capture: Read a paragraph, verse or small section	
Reflect: Focus on the small section and write it down.	
Unite: Write down those 3 - 5 words in the section to activate the brain. Write them 3 times	
Silence: Take 5 minutes to go inside and then write you observations about what you learned.	
Healthy Acts: How did I use and implement the passage I reflected upon today?	

Daily Crush: Day 10

Capture: Read a paragraph, verse or small section	
Reflect: Focus on the small section and write it down.	
Unite: Write down those 3 - 5 words in the section to activate the brain. Write them 3 times	
Silence: Take 5 minutes to go inside and then write you observations about what you learned.	
Healthy Acts: How did I use and implement the passage I reflected upon today?	

Daily Crush: Day 11

Capture: Read a paragraph, verse or small section	
Reflect: Focus on the small section and write it down.	
Unite: Write down those 3 - 5 words in the section to activate the brain. Write them 3 times	
Silence: Take 5 minutes to go inside and then write you observations about what you learned.	
Healthy Acts: How did I use and implement the passage I reflected upon today?	

Daily Crush: Day 12

Capture: Read a paragraph, verse or small section	
Reflect: Focus on the small section and write it down.	
Unite: Write down those 3 - 5 words in the section to activate the brain. Write them 3 times	
Silence: Take 5 minutes to go inside and then write you observations about what you learned.	
Healthy Acts: How did I use and implement the passage I reflected upon today?	

Daily Crush: Day 13

Capture: Read a paragraph, verse or small section	
Reflect: Focus on the small section and write it down.	
Unite: Write down those 3 - 5 words in the section to activate the brain. Write them 3 times	
Silence: Take 5 minutes to go inside and then write you observations about what you learned.	
Healthy Acts: How did I use and implement the passage I reflected upon today?	

Daily Crush: Day 14

Capture: Read a paragraph, verse or small section	
Reflect: Focus on the small section and write it down.	
Unite: Write down those 3 - 5 words in the section to activate the brain. Write them 3 times	
Silence: Take 5 minutes to go inside and then write you observations about what you learned.	
Healthy Acts: How did I use and implement the passage I reflected upon today?	

WEEK 2 WEEKLY WARRIORS

Random Act of Kindness:	
Anticipation:	
Expectation:	
Results:	

Daily Crush: Day 15

Capture: Read a paragraph, verse or small section	
Reflect: Focus on the small section and write it down.	
Unite: Write down those 3 - 5 words in the section to activate the brain. Write them 3 times	
Silence: Take 5 minutes to go inside and then write you observations about what you learned.	
Healthy Acts: How did I use and implement the passage I reflected upon today?	

Daily Crush: Day 16

Capture: Read a paragraph, verse or small section	
Reflect: Focus on the small section and write it down.	
Unite: Write down those 3 - 5 words in the section to activate the brain. Write them 3 times	
Silence: Take 5 minutes to go inside and then write you observations about what you learned.	
Healthy Acts: How did I use and implement the passage I reflected upon today?	

Daily Crush: Day 17

Capture: Read a paragraph, verse or small section	
Reflect: Focus on the small section and write it down.	
Unite: Write down those 3 - 5 words in the section to activate the brain. Write them 3 times	
Silence: Take 5 minutes to go inside and then write you observations about what you learned.	
Healthy Acts: How did I use and implement the passage I reflected upon today?	

Daily Crush: Day 18

Capture: Read a paragraph, verse or small section	
Reflect: Focus on the small section and write it down.	
Unite: Write down those 3 - 5 words in the section to activate the brain. Write them 3 times	
Silence: Take 5 minutes to go inside and then write you observations about what you learned.	
Healthy Acts: How did I use and implement the passage I reflected upon today?	

Daily Crush: Day 19

Capture: Read a paragraph, verse or small section	
Reflect: Focus on the small section and write it down.	
Unite: Write down those 3 - 5 words in the section to activate the brain. Write them 3 times	
Silence: Take 5 minutes to go inside and then write you observations about what you learned.	
Healthy Acts: How did I use and implement the passage I reflected upon today?	

Daily Crush: Day 20

Capture: Read a paragraph, verse or small section	
Reflect: Focus on the small section and write it down.	
Unite: Write down those 3 - 5 words in the section to activate the brain. Write them 3 times	
Silence: Take 5 minutes to go inside and then write you observations about what you learned.	
Healthy Acts: How did I use and implement the passage I reflected upon today?	

Daily Crush: Day 21

Capture: Read a paragraph, verse or small section	
Reflect: Focus on the small section and write it down.	
Unite: Write down those 3 - 5 words in the section to activate the brain. Write them 3 times	
Silence: Take 5 minutes to go inside and then write you observations about what you learned.	
Healthy Acts: How did I use and implement the passage I reflected upon today?	

WEEK 3: WEEKLY WARRIORS

Random Act of Kindness:	
Anticipation:	
Results:	
Expectation:	

Daily Crush; Day 22

Capture: Read a paragraph, verse or small section	
Reflect: Focus on the small section and write it down.	
Unite: Write down those 3 - 5 words in the section to activate the brain. Write them 3 times	
Silence: Take 5 minutes to go inside and then write you observations about what you learned.	
Healthy Acts: How did I use and implement the passage I reflected upon today?	

Daily Crush; Day 23

Capture: Read a paragraph, verse or small section	
Reflect: Focus on the small section and write it down.	
Unite: Write down those 3 - 5 words in the section to activate the brain. Write them 3 times	
Silence: Take 5 minutes to go inside and then write you observations about what you learned.	
Healthy Acts: How did I use and implement the passage I reflected upon today?	

Daily Crush: Day 24

Capture: Read a paragraph, verse or small section	
Reflect: Focus on the small section and write it down.	
Unite: Write down those 3 - 5 words in the section to activate the brain. Write them 3 times	
Silence: Take 5 minutes to go inside and then write you observations about what you learned.	
Healthy Acts: How did I use and implement the passage I reflected upon today?	

Daily Crush: Day 25

Capture: Read a paragraph, verse or small section	
Reflect: Focus on the small section and write it down.	
Unite: Write down those 3 - 5 words in the section to activate the brain. Write them 3 times	
Silence: Take 5 minutes to go inside and then write you observations about what you learned.	
Healthy Acts: How did I use and implement the passage I reflected upon today?	

Daily Crush: Day 26

Capture: Read a paragraph, verse or small section	
Reflect: Focus on the small section and write it down.	
Unite: Write down those 3 - 5 words in the section to activate the brain. Write them 3 times	
Silence: Take 5 minutes to go inside and then write you observations about what you learned.	
Healthy Acts: How did I use and implement the passage I reflected upon today?	

Daily Crush: Day 27

Capture: Read a paragraph, verse or small section	
Reflect: Focus on the small section and write it down.	
Unite: Write down those 3 - 5 words in the section to activate the brain. Write them 3 times	
Silence: Take 5 minutes to go inside and then write you observations about what you learned.	
Healthy Acts: How did I use and implement the passage I reflected upon today?	

Daily Crush: Day 28

Capture: Read a paragraph, verse or small section	
Reflect: Focus on the small section and write it down.	
Unite: Write down those 3 - 5 words in the section to activate the brain. Write them 3 times	
Silence: Take 5 minutes to go inside and then write you observations about what you learned.	
Healthy Acts: How did I use and implement the passage I reflected upon today?	

Congratulations! You have completed your 28 days.
You can get to decide if you want to do this for a lifetime!

WEEK 4 WEEKLY WARRIORS

Random Act of Kindness:	
Anticipation:	
Expectation:	
Results:	

Congratulations! You have completed your 4 weeks.

You can get to decide if you want to do this for a lifetime!

FOOD SENSITIVITY TESTING

The purpose of the detox is to not only rid your body of toxins, but to educate you on how your body is designed to eat and process food. Enjoy your new way of eating, this is a part of your lifestyle now. Drink plenty of pure water and include nutritionally rich foods. Love and care for your body and it will respond accordingly. You have come a long way and laid the foundation to the new YOU, great job! Let's keep the momentum, and if you have any questions, ask!

How to: In the reintroduction or food-challenge phase, you should add one food group at a time back into your diet every three days, ensuring use of organic, grass fed, pasture raised, GMO-free foods to identify reactions or sensitivities to the actual food itself instead of possible additive sensitivities.

Introduce one new food, every 4th day. Most food reactions are delayed and may be experienced up to 4 days after the offending food was eaten, for example:

Day 1- you may choose to introduce eggs, so enjoy a big omelet

Day 2 and 3- you will omit eggs and if you notice symptoms or reactions such as gas, bloating, heartburn, upset stomach, brain fog, headache, sleepiness, skin breakouts etc. write them down in this booklet. You will want to omit them from your diet due to the reactions you had.

Day 4- you will move onto the next food, tomatoes for example, you should have a large quantity of tomatoes and on

Day 5 and 6- do not eat any tomatoes

Day 7- if you have no reaction, you may eat them freely and the next food can be introduced. Please continue with this pattern until all the foods listed above have been re-introduced. You may choose to skip certain foods if you do not enjoy them and/or already know you have a sensitivity. When reintroducing foods after this program PLEASE be aware that there are certain foods that may not create symptoms or visible signs of distress, even though they trigger immune reactions and intestinal inflammation. These are hidden health destroyers such as gluten, dairy, coffee, and others.

While on the reintroduction phase you will be back on the eating plan from week 2 of the detox. No supplements are necessary at this point

For the next 21 – 27 days, keep a food journal of what you eat. It is very important to "feed" your body good whole foods on a consistent basis (3-4x/day). Your body needs the appropriate caloric intake daily for your metabolism to work to optimum levels. You should now know that weight loss is not as simple as calories in-calories out. Many patients do not eat enough

Tomatoes (organic preferred)
Serving(s) Size _____
How Do I feel?

_____
_____
_____

Peppers (organic, bell, chili, paprika etc.)
Serving(s) Size _____
How Do I feel?

_____
_____
_____

Egg Plant (organic, preferred)

Serving(s) Size _____

How Do I feel?

_____

_____

_____

Potatoes (organic, red, yellow, white potatoes)

Serving(s) Size _____

How Do I feel?

_____

_____

_____

Eggs (organic, free range, pasture)

Serving(s) Size _____

How Do I feel?

_____

_____

_____

Nuts and seeds (organic, raw, roasted, sprouted)

Serving(s) Size _____

How Do I feel?

_____

_____

_____

Coffee (Organic, Fair Trade, caffeinated)

Serving(s) Size _____

How Do I feel?

_____

_____

_____

Milk (organic, cow, cream or half and half)
Serving(s) Size _____

How Do I feel?

_____

_____

_____

Yogurt (organic goat, cow, kefir)
Serving(s) Size _____
How Do I feel?

_____

_____

_____

Cheese (organic, goat, cow)
Serving(s) Size _____
How Do I feel?

_____

_____

_____

Red Meat (Grass fed, bison, beef preferred)
Serving(s) Size _____

How Do I feel?

_____

_____

_____

Pork (no nitrates, bacon, sausage etc.)

Serving(s) Size _____

How Do I feel?

_____

_____

_____

Corn (organic, sprouted preferred)

Serving(s) Size _____

How Do I feel?

_____

_____

_____

Wheat, Grains (organic, sprouted preferred)

Serving(s) Size _____

How Do I feel?

_____

_____

_____

Other (Legumes, ...etc.)

Serving(s) Size _____

How Do I feel?

_____

_____

_____

Made in the USA
Columbia, SC
22 July 2021